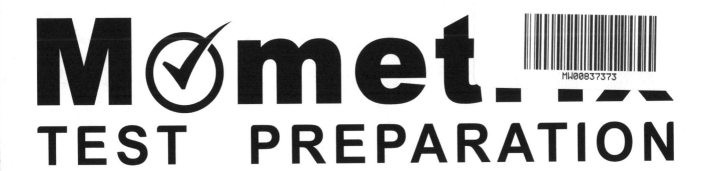

CPSGT

Exam Secrets Study Guide

DEAR FUTURE EXAM SUCCESS STORY

First of all, **THANK YOU** for purchasing Mometrix study materials!

Second, congratulations! You are one of the few determined test-takers who are committed to doing whatever it takes to excel on your exam. **You have come to the right place.** We developed these study materials with one goal in mind: to deliver you the information you need in a format that's concise and easy to use.

In addition to optimizing your guide for the content of the test, we've outlined our recommended steps for breaking down the preparation process into small, attainable goals so you can make sure you stay on track.

We've also analyzed the entire test-taking process, identifying the most common pitfalls and showing how you can overcome them and be ready for any curveball the test throws you.

Standardized testing is one of the biggest obstacles on your road to success, which only increases the importance of doing well in the high-pressure, high-stakes environment of test day. Your results on this test could have a significant impact on your future, and this guide provides the information and practical advice to help you achieve your full potential on test day.

Your success is our success

We would love to hear from you! If you would like to share the story of your exam success or if you have any questions or comments in regard to our products, please contact us at **800-673-8175** or **support@mometrix.com**.

Thanks again for your business and we wish you continued success!

Sincerely,
The Mometrix Test Preparation Team

> **Need more help? Check out our flashcards at:**
> **http://mometrixflashcards.com/RPSGT**

TABLE OF CONTENTS

Introduction

Thank you for purchasing this resource! You have made the choice to prepare yourself for a test that could have a huge impact on your future, and this guide is designed to help you be fully ready for test day. Obviously, it's important to have a solid understanding of the test material, but you also need to be prepared for the unique environment and stressors of the test, so that you can perform to the best of your abilities.

For this purpose, the first section that appears in this guide is the **Secret Keys**. We've devoted countless hours to meticulously researching what works and what doesn't, and we've boiled down our findings to the five most impactful steps you can take to improve your performance on the test. We start at the beginning with study planning and move through the preparation process, all the way to the testing strategies that will help you get the most out of what you know when you're finally sitting in front of the test.

We recommend that you start preparing for your test as far in advance as possible. However, if you've bought this guide as a last-minute study resource and only have a few days before your test, we recommend that you skip over the first two Secret Keys since they address a long-term study plan.

If you struggle with **test anxiety**, we strongly encourage you to check out our recommendations for how you can overcome it. Test anxiety is a formidable foe, but it can be beaten, and we want to make sure you have the tools you need to defeat it.

1

Secret Key #1 – Plan Big, Study Small

There's a lot riding on your performance. If you want to ace this test, you're going to need to keep your skills sharp and the material fresh in your mind. You need a plan that lets you review everything you need to know while still fitting in your schedule. We'll break this strategy down into three categories.

Information Organization

Start with the information you already have: the official test outline. From this, you can make a complete list of all the concepts you need to cover before the test. Organize these concepts into groups that can be studied together, and create a list of any related vocabulary you need to learn so you can brush up on any difficult terms. You'll want to keep this vocabulary list handy once you actually start studying since you may need to add to it along the way.

Time Management

Once you have your set of study concepts, decide how to spread them out over the time you have left before the test. Break your study plan into small, clear goals so you have a manageable task for each day and know exactly what you're doing. Then just focus on one small step at a time. When you manage your time this way, you don't need to spend hours at a time studying. Studying a small block of content for a short period each day helps you retain information better and avoid stressing over how much you have left to do. You can relax knowing that you have a plan to cover everything in time. In order for this strategy to be effective though, you have to start studying early and stick to your schedule. Avoid the exhaustion and futility that comes from last-minute cramming!

Study Environment

The environment you study in has a big impact on your learning. Studying in a coffee shop, while probably more enjoyable, is not likely to be as fruitful as studying in a quiet room. It's important to keep distractions to a minimum. You're only planning to study for a short block of time, so make the most of it. Don't pause to check your phone or get up to find a snack. It's also important to **avoid multitasking**. Research has consistently shown that multitasking will make your studying dramatically less effective. Your study area should also be comfortable and well-lit so you don't have the distraction of straining your eyes or sitting on an uncomfortable chair.

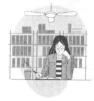 The time of day you study is also important. You want to be rested and alert. Don't wait until just before bedtime. Study when you'll be most likely to comprehend and remember. Even better, if you know what time of day your test will be, set that time aside for study. That way your brain will be used to working on that subject at that specific time and you'll have a better chance of recalling information.

Finally, it can be helpful to team up with others who are studying for the same test. Your actual studying should be done in as isolated an environment as possible, but the work of organizing the information and setting up the study plan can be divided up. In between study sessions, you can discuss with your teammates the concepts that you're all studying and quiz each other on the details. Just be sure that your teammates are as serious about the test as you are. If you find that your study time is being replaced with social time, you might need to find a new team.

2

Secret Key #2 – Make Your Studying Count

You're devoting a lot of time and effort to preparing for this test, so you want to be absolutely certain it will pay off. This means doing more than just reading the content and hoping you can remember it on test day. It's important to make every minute of study count. There are two main areas you can focus on to make your studying count.

Retention

It doesn't matter how much time you study if you can't remember the material. You need to make sure you are retaining the concepts. To check your retention of the information you're learning, try recalling it at later times with minimal prompting. Try carrying around flashcards and glance at one or two from time to time or ask a friend who's also studying for the test to quiz you.

To enhance your retention, look for ways to put the information into practice so that you can apply it rather than simply recalling it. If you're using the information in practical ways, it will be much easier to remember. Similarly, it helps to solidify a concept in your mind if you're not only reading it to yourself but also explaining it to someone else. Ask a friend to let you teach them about a concept you're a little shaky on (or speak aloud to an imaginary audience if necessary). As you try to summarize, define, give examples, and answer your friend's questions, you'll understand the concepts better and they will stay with you longer. Finally, step back for a big picture view and ask yourself how each piece of information fits with the whole subject. When you link the different concepts together and see them working together as a whole, it's easier to remember the individual components.

Finally, practice showing your work on any multi-step problems, even if you're just studying. Writing out each step you take to solve a problem will help solidify the process in your mind, and you'll be more likely to remember it during the test.

Modality

Modality simply refers to the means or method by which you study. Choosing a study modality that fits your own individual learning style is crucial. No two people learn best in exactly the same way, so it's important to know your strengths and use them to your advantage.

For example, if you learn best by visualization, focus on visualizing a concept in your mind and draw an image or a diagram. Try color-coding your notes, illustrating them, or creating symbols that will trigger your mind to recall a learned concept. If you learn best by hearing or discussing information, find a study partner who learns the same way or read aloud to yourself. Think about how to put the information in your own words. Imagine that you are giving a lecture on the topic and record yourself so you can listen to it later.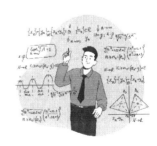

For any learning style, flashcards can be helpful. Organize the information so you can take advantage of spare moments to review. Underline key words or phrases. Use different colors for different categories. Mnemonic devices (such as creating a short list in which every item starts with the same letter) can also help with retention. Find what works best for you and use it to store the information in your mind most effectively and easily.

3

Secret Key #3 – Practice the Right Way

Your success on test day depends not only on how many hours you put into preparing, but also on whether you prepared the right way. It's good to check along the way to see if your studying is paying off. One of the most effective ways to do this is by taking practice tests to evaluate your progress. Practice tests are useful because they show exactly where you need to improve. Every time you take a practice test, pay special attention to these three groups of questions:

- The questions you got wrong
- The questions you had to guess on, even if you guessed right
- The questions you found difficult or slow to work through

This will show you exactly what your weak areas are, and where you need to devote more study time. Ask yourself why each of these questions gave you trouble. Was it because you didn't understand the material? Was it because you didn't remember the vocabulary? Do you need more repetitions on this type of question to build speed and confidence? Dig into those questions and figure out how you can strengthen your weak areas as you go back to review the material.

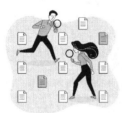 Additionally, many practice tests have a section explaining the answer choices. It can be tempting to read the explanation and think that you now have a good understanding of the concept. However, an explanation likely only covers part of the question's broader context. Even if the explanation makes perfect sense, **go back and investigate** every concept related to the question until you're positive you have a thorough understanding.

As you go along, keep in mind that the practice test is just that: practice. Memorizing these questions and answers will not be very helpful on the actual test because it is unlikely to have any of the same exact questions. If you only know the right answers to the sample questions, you won't be prepared for the real thing. **Study the concepts** until you understand them fully, and then you'll be able to answer any question that shows up on the test.

It's important to wait on the practice tests until you're ready. If you take a test on your first day of study, you may be overwhelmed by the amount of material covered and how much you need to learn. Work up to it gradually.

On test day, you'll need to be prepared for answering questions, managing your time, and using the test-taking strategies you've learned. It's a lot to balance, like a mental marathon that will have a big impact on your future. Like training for a marathon, you'll need to start slowly and work your way up. When test day arrives, you'll be ready.

Start with the strategies you've read in the first two Secret Keys—plan your course and study in the way that works best for you. If you have time, consider using multiple study resources to get different approaches to the same concepts. It can be helpful to see difficult concepts from more than one angle. Then find a good source for practice tests. Many times, the test website will suggest potential study resources or provide sample tests.

Practice Test Strategy

If you're able to find at least three practice tests, we recommend this strategy:

UNTIMED AND OPEN-BOOK PRACTICE

Take the first test with no time constraints and with your notes and study guide handy. Take your time and focus on applying the strategies you've learned.

TIMED AND OPEN-BOOK PRACTICE

Take the second practice test open-book as well, but set a timer and practice pacing yourself to finish in time.

TIMED AND CLOSED-BOOK PRACTICE

Take any other practice tests as if it were test day. Set a timer and put away your study materials. Sit at a table or desk in a quiet room, imagine yourself at the testing center, and answer questions as quickly and accurately as possible.

Keep repeating timed and closed-book tests on a regular basis until you run out of practice tests or it's time for the actual test. Your mind will be ready for the schedule and stress of test day, and you'll be able to focus on recalling the material you've learned.

Secret Key #4 – Pace Yourself

Once you're fully prepared for the material on the test, your biggest challenge on test day will be managing your time. Just knowing that the clock is ticking can make you panic even if you have plenty of time left. Work on pacing yourself so you can build confidence against the time constraints of the exam. Pacing is a difficult skill to master, especially in a high-pressure environment, so **practice is vital**.

Set time expectations for your pace based on how much time is available. For example, if a section has 60 questions and the time limit is 30 minutes, you know you have to average 30 seconds or less per question in order to answer them all. Although 30 seconds is the hard limit, set 25 seconds per question as your goal, so you reserve extra time to spend on harder questions. When you budget extra time for the harder questions, you no longer have any reason to stress when those questions take longer to answer.

Don't let this time expectation distract you from working through the test at a calm, steady pace, but keep it in mind so you don't spend too much time on any one question. Recognize that taking extra time on one question you don't understand may keep you from answering two that you do understand later in the test. If your time limit for a question is up and you're still not sure of the answer, mark it and move on, and come back to it later if the time and the test format allow. If the testing format doesn't allow you to return to earlier questions, just make an educated guess; then put it out of your mind and move on.

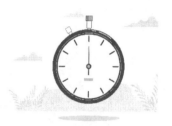

On the easier questions, be careful not to rush. It may seem wise to hurry through them so you have more time for the challenging ones, but it's not worth missing one if you know the concept and just didn't take the time to read the question fully. Work efficiently but make sure you understand the question and have looked at all of the answer choices, since more than one may seem right at first.

Even if you're paying attention to the time, you may find yourself a little behind at some point. You should speed up to get back on track, but do so wisely. Don't panic; just take a few seconds less on each question until you're caught up. Don't guess without thinking, but do look through the answer choices and eliminate any you know are wrong. If you can get down to two choices, it is often worthwhile to guess from those. Once you've chosen an answer, move on and don't dwell on any that you skipped or had to hurry through. If a question was taking too long, chances are it was one of the harder ones, so you weren't as likely to get it right anyway.

On the other hand, if you find yourself getting ahead of schedule, it may be beneficial to slow down a little. The more quickly you work, the more likely you are to make a careless mistake that will affect your score. You've budgeted time for each question, so don't be afraid to spend that time. Practice an efficient but careful pace to get the most out of the time you have.

Secret Key #5 – Have a Plan for Guessing

When you're taking the test, you may find yourself stuck on a question. Some of the answer choices seem better than others, but you don't see the one answer choice that is obviously correct. What do you do?

The scenario described above is very common, yet most test takers have not effectively prepared for it. Developing and practicing a plan for guessing may be one of the single most effective uses of your time as you get ready for the exam.

In developing your plan for guessing, there are three questions to address:

- When should you start the guessing process?
- How should you narrow down the choices?
- Which answer should you choose?

When to Start the Guessing Process

Unless your plan for guessing is to select C every time (which, despite its merits, is not what we recommend), you need to leave yourself enough time to apply your answer elimination strategies. Since you have a limited amount of time for each question, that means that if you're going to give yourself the best shot at guessing correctly, you have to decide quickly whether or not you will guess.

Of course, the best-case scenario is that you don't have to guess at all, so first, see if you can answer the question based on your knowledge of the subject and basic reasoning skills. Focus on the key words in the question and try to jog your memory of related topics. Give yourself a chance to bring the knowledge to mind, but once you realize that you don't have (or you can't access) the knowledge you need to answer the question, it's time to start the guessing process.

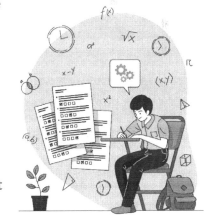

It's almost always better to start the guessing process too early than too late. It only takes a few seconds to remember something and answer the question from knowledge. Carefully eliminating wrong answer choices takes longer. Plus, going through the process of eliminating answer choices can actually help jog your memory.

Summary: Start the guessing process as soon as you decide that you can't answer the question based on your knowledge.

How to Narrow Down the Choices

The next chapter in this book (**Test-Taking Strategies**) includes a wide range of strategies for how to approach questions and how to look for answer choices to eliminate. You will definitely want to read those carefully, practice them, and figure out which ones work best for you. Here though, we're going to address a mindset rather than a particular strategy.

Your odds of guessing an answer correctly depend on how many options you are choosing from.

Number of options left	5	4	3	2	1
Odds of guessing correctly	20%	25%	33%	50%	100%

You can see from this chart just how valuable it is to be able to eliminate incorrect answers and make an educated guess, but there are two things that many test takers do that cause them to miss out on the benefits of guessing:

- Accidentally eliminating the correct answer
- Selecting an answer based on an impression

We'll look at the first one here, and the second one in the next section.

To avoid accidentally eliminating the correct answer, we recommend a thought exercise called **the $5 challenge**. In this challenge, you only eliminate an answer choice from contention if you are willing to bet $5 on it being wrong. Why $5? Five dollars is a small but not insignificant amount of money. It's an amount you could afford to lose but wouldn't want to throw away. And while losing

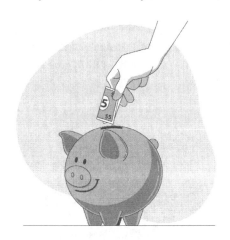

$5 once might not hurt too much, doing it twenty times will set you back $100. In the same way, each small decision you make—eliminating a choice here, guessing on a question there—won't by itself impact your score very much, but when you put them all together, they can make a big difference. By holding each answer choice elimination decision to a higher standard, you can reduce the risk of accidentally eliminating the correct answer.

The $5 challenge can also be applied in a positive sense: If you are willing to bet $5 that an answer choice *is* correct, go ahead and mark it as correct.

Summary: Only eliminate an answer choice if you are willing to bet $5 that it is wrong.

8

Which Answer to Choose

You're taking the test. You've run into a hard question and decided you'll have to guess. You've eliminated all the answer choices you're willing to bet $5 on. Now you have to pick an answer. Why do we even need to talk about this? Why can't you just pick whichever one you feel like when the time comes?

The answer to these questions is that if you don't come into the test with a plan, you'll rely on your impression to select an answer choice, and if you do that, you risk falling into a trap. The test writers know that everyone who takes their test will be guessing on some of the questions, so they intentionally write wrong answer choices to seem plausible. You still have to pick an answer though, and if the wrong answer choices are designed to look right, how can you ever be sure that you're not falling for their trap? The best solution we've found to this dilemma is to take the decision out of your hands entirely. Here is the process we recommend:

Once you've eliminated any choices that you are confident (willing to bet $5) are wrong, select the first remaining choice as your answer.

Whether you choose to select the first remaining choice, the second, or the last, the important thing is that you use some preselected standard. Using this approach guarantees that you will not be enticed into selecting an answer choice that looks right, because you are not basing your decision on how the answer choices look.

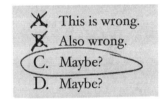

This is not meant to make you question your knowledge. Instead, it is to help you recognize the difference between your knowledge and your impressions. There's a huge difference between thinking an answer is right because of what you know, and thinking an answer is right because it looks or sounds like it should be right.

Summary: To ensure that your selection is appropriately random, make a predetermined selection from among all answer choices you have not eliminated.

Test-Taking Strategies

This section contains a list of test-taking strategies that you may find helpful as you work through the test. By taking what you know and applying logical thought, you can maximize your chances of answering any question correctly!

It is very important to realize that every question is different and every person is different: no single strategy will work on every question, and no single strategy will work for every person. That's why we've included all of them here, so you can try them out and determine which ones work best for different types of questions and which ones work best for you.

Question Strategies

⊘ READ CAREFULLY

Read the question and the answer choices carefully. Don't miss the question because you misread the terms. You have plenty of time to read each question thoroughly and make sure you understand what is being asked. Yet a happy medium must be attained, so don't waste too much time. You must read carefully and efficiently.

⊘ CONTEXTUAL CLUES

Look for contextual clues. If the question includes a word you are not familiar with, look at the immediate context for some indication of what the word might mean. Contextual clues can often give you all the information you need to decipher the meaning of an unfamiliar word. Even if you can't determine the meaning, you may be able to narrow down the possibilities enough to make a solid guess at the answer to the question.

⊘ PREFIXES

If you're having trouble with a word in the question or answer choices, try dissecting it. Take advantage of every clue that the word might include. Prefixes can be a huge help. Usually, they allow you to determine a basic meaning. *Pre-* means before, *post-* means after, *pro-* is positive, *de-* is negative. From prefixes, you can get an idea of the general meaning of the word and try to put it into context.

⊘ HEDGE WORDS

Watch out for critical hedge words, such as *likely, may, can, sometimes, often, almost, mostly, usually, generally, rarely,* and *sometimes.* Question writers insert these hedge phrases to cover every possibility. Often an answer choice will be wrong simply because it leaves no room for exception. Be on guard for answer choices that have definitive words such as *exactly* and *always.*

⊘ SWITCHBACK WORDS

Stay alert for *switchbacks.* These are the words and phrases frequently used to alert you to shifts in thought. The most common switchback words are *but, although,* and *however.* Others include *nevertheless, on the other hand, even though, while, in spite of, despite,* and *regardless of.* Switchback words are important to catch because they can change the direction of the question or an answer choice.

⊘ Face Value

When in doubt, use common sense. Accept the situation in the problem at face value. Don't read too much into it. These problems will not require you to make wild assumptions. If you have to go beyond creativity and warp time or space in order to have an answer choice fit the question, then you should move on and consider the other answer choices. These are normal problems rooted in reality. The applicable relationship or explanation may not be readily apparent, but it is there for you to figure out. Use your common sense to interpret anything that isn't clear.

Answer Choice Strategies

⊘ Answer Selection

The most thorough way to pick an answer choice is to identify and eliminate wrong answers until only one is left, then confirm it is the correct answer. Sometimes an answer choice may immediately seem right, but be careful. The test writers will usually put more than one reasonable answer choice on each question, so take a second to read all of them and make sure that the other choices are not equally obvious. As long as you have time left, it is better to read every answer choice than to pick the first one that looks right without checking the others.

⊘ Answer Choice Families

An answer choice family consists of two (in rare cases, three) answer choices that are very similar in construction and cannot all be true at the same time. If you see two answer choices that are direct opposites or parallels, one of them is usually the correct answer. For instance, if one answer choice says that quantity x increases and another either says that quantity x decreases (opposite) or says that quantity y increases (parallel), then those answer choices would fall into the same family. An answer choice that doesn't match the construction of the answer choice family is more likely to be incorrect. Most questions will not have answer choice families, but when they do appear, you should be prepared to recognize them.

⊘ Eliminate Answers

Eliminate answer choices as soon as you realize they are wrong, but make sure you consider all possibilities. If you are eliminating answer choices and realize that the last one you are left with is also wrong, don't panic. Start over and consider each choice again. There may be something you missed the first time that you will realize on the second pass.

⊘ Avoid Fact Traps

Don't be distracted by an answer choice that is factually true but doesn't answer the question. You are looking for the choice that answers the question. Stay focused on what the question is asking for so you don't accidentally pick an answer that is true but incorrect. Always go back to the question and make sure the answer choice you've selected actually answers the question and is not merely a true statement.

⊘ Extreme Statements

In general, you should avoid answers that put forth extreme actions as standard practice or proclaim controversial ideas as established fact. An answer choice that states the "process should be used in certain situations, if…" is much more likely to be correct than one that states the "process should be discontinued completely." The first is a calm rational statement and doesn't even make a definitive, uncompromising stance, using a hedge word *if* to provide wiggle room, whereas the second choice is far more extreme.

11

⊘ BENCHMARK

As you read through the answer choices and you come across one that seems to answer the question well, mentally select that answer choice. This is not your final answer, but it's the one that will help you evaluate the other answer choices. The one that you selected is your benchmark or standard for judging each of the other answer choices. Every other answer choice must be compared to your benchmark. That choice is correct until proven otherwise by another answer choice beating it. If you find a better answer, then that one becomes your new benchmark. Once you've decided that no other choice answers the question as well as your benchmark, you have your final answer.

⊘ PREDICT THE ANSWER

Before you even start looking at the answer choices, it is often best to try to predict the answer. When you come up with the answer on your own, it is easier to avoid distractions and traps because you will know exactly what to look for. The right answer choice is unlikely to be word-for-word what you came up with, but it should be a close match. Even if you are confident that you have the right answer, you should still take the time to read each option before moving on.

General Strategies

⊘ TOUGH QUESTIONS

If you are stumped on a problem or it appears too hard or too difficult, don't waste time. Move on! Remember though, if you can quickly check for obviously incorrect answer choices, your chances of guessing correctly are greatly improved. Before you completely give up, at least try to knock out a couple of possible answers. Eliminate what you can and then guess at the remaining answer choices before moving on.

⊘ CHECK YOUR WORK

Since you will probably not know every term listed and the answer to every question, it is important that you get credit for the ones that you do know. Don't miss any questions through careless mistakes. If at all possible, try to take a second to look back over your answer selection and make sure you've selected the correct answer choice and haven't made a costly careless mistake (such as marking an answer choice that you didn't mean to mark). This quick double check should more than pay for itself in caught mistakes for the time it costs.

⊘ PACE YOURSELF

It's easy to be overwhelmed when you're looking at a page full of questions; your mind is confused and full of random thoughts, and the clock is ticking down faster than you would like. Calm down and maintain the pace that you have set for yourself. Especially as you get down to the last few minutes of the test, don't let the small numbers on the clock make you panic. As long as you are on track by monitoring your pace, you are guaranteed to have time for each question.

⊘ DON'T RUSH

It is very easy to make errors when you are in a hurry. Maintaining a fast pace in answering questions is pointless if it makes you miss questions that you would have gotten right otherwise. Test writers like to include distracting information and wrong answers that seem right. Taking a little extra time to avoid careless mistakes can make all the difference in your test score. Find a pace that allows you to be confident in the answers that you select.

⊘ Keep Moving

Panicking will not help you pass the test, so do your best to stay calm and keep moving. Taking deep breaths and going through the answer elimination steps you practiced can help to break through a stress barrier and keep your pace.

Final Notes

The combination of a solid foundation of content knowledge and the confidence that comes from practicing your plan for applying that knowledge is the key to maximizing your performance on test day. As your foundation of content knowledge is built up and strengthened, you'll find that the strategies included in this chapter become more and more effective in helping you quickly sift through the distractions and traps of the test to isolate the correct answer.

Now that you're preparing to move forward into the test content chapters of this book, be sure to keep your goal in mind. As you read, think about how you will be able to apply this information on the test. If you've already seen sample questions for the test and you have an idea of the question format and style, try to come up with questions of your own that you can answer based on what you're reading. This will give you valuable practice applying your knowledge in the same ways you can expect to on test day.

Good luck and good studying!

Sleep Study Preparation and Performance

Patient Information and Clinical Assessment

COMMON ABBREVIATIONS FOR SLEEP TECHNOLOGY

Common abbreviations used for sleep technology include the following:

Abbreviation	Meaning	Abbreviation	Meaning
AI	Apnea index	RBD	REM behavior disorder
AHI	Apnea-hypopnea index	RDI	Respiratory disturbance index
CAP	Cyclic alternating pattern	REM	Rapid eye movement
EDS	Excessive daytime sleepiness	RERA	Respiratory effort-related arousals
EPAP	Expiratory positive airway pressure	RLS	Restless legs syndrome
IEA	Interictal epileptiform activity	SAH	Sleep apnea-hypopnea
IPAP	Inspiratory positive airway pressure	SE	Sleep efficiency
Non-REM	Non-rapid eye movement	SOL	Sleep onset latency
OA	Obstructive apnea	SWS	Short-wave sleep
OH	Obstructive hypopnea	SPT	Sleep period time
OSAS	Obstructive sleep apnea syndrome	TST	Total sleep time
OSA/H	Obstructive sleep apnea-hypopnea	TSP	Total sleep period
PLMS	Periodic limb movements in sleep	TWT	Total wake time
PRC	Phase response curve	WASO	Wake-after-sleep onset
PSG	Polysomnogram		

PROCEDURE ORDERS

Procedure orders are usually generated by the attending physician and are explicit about the type of testing, including any special orders to accommodate special needs, such as for the patient with dementia or diabetes. They must be signed and dated. Orders include any routine medications the patient takes before or during the test. Since most states do not allow sleep technicians to administer medications, medications are either self-administered, or other licensed staff is available to administer them. Technicians must be aware of the medications taken by the patient in the event the patient terminates the testing and leaves the facility, which may put the patient or others in danger, if, for example, the patient has taken sleeping medication. The procedure orders are checked in relation to the patient questionnaire to resolve any discrepancies, and the physician is contacted if necessary.

IMPORTANCE OF VERIFYING CLINICIAN ORDERS PRIOR TO IMPLEMENTATION

A sleep study requires an order from a medical provider. This order should include the type of sleep study to be performed along with an ordering diagnosis. It is very important to carefully review the order to ensure that the correct study and any specific testing requests are performed. Following

15

results of the sleep study, orders should be written for the type of therapy recommended to treat the patient's sleep apnea. These should also be reviewed carefully to ensure the proper equipment (mask, nasal device, etc.) is ordered and fit for the patient. Any details regarding the specific settings for CPAP or BiPAP therapy should also be noted to ensure the patient is receiving the appropriate amount of positive airway pressure to treat their sleep apnea. If a trial of the device is to be performed, such as a PAP-Nap trial, this should also be indicated on the orders. All details of the orders for the patient should always be carefully reviewed to ensure that appropriate testing and treatment are offered to the patient.

PATIENT'S HISTORY AND PHYSICAL

The history and physical is reviewed by the technician before the first meeting with the patient, if possible, as this information can guide the initial assessment as well as the evaluation during and after the testing.

Sleep disorders	Obstructive/central sleep apnea, narcolepsy, circadian rhythm disorders, restless legs syndrome, periodic leg movement, parasomnias, and insomnia
Respiratory disorders	Chronic obstructive pulmonary disease, cystic fibrosis, restrictive lung diseases, and asthma
Neuromuscular diseases	Multiple sclerosis, amyotrophic lateral sclerosis, myasthenia gravis, poliomyelitis, and myotonic dystrophy
Spinal cord injury	Bilateral diaphragmatic paralysis
Gastrointestinal disorders	Gastroesophageal reflux disease and functional bowel disorders
Endocrine disorders	Hypothyroidism, acromegaly, Cushing's syndrome, Addison's disease, diabetes mellitus, and diabetes insipidus.
Rheumatologic disorders	Pain syndromes and fibromyalgia
Kidney/urinary disorders	End-stage renal disease and urinary frequency
Infectious diseases	HIV/AIDS, Lyme disease, and human African trypanosomiasis
Cardiovascular disorders	Heart block, dysrhythmias, congestive heart failure, coronary artery disease, and atrial fibrillation
Psychiatric disorders	Bipolar disorder, depression, post-traumatic stress disorder, and schizophrenia

ESTABLISHING BASELINES FOR NEW PATIENTS

Prior to initiating sleep study interventions there are critical steps that the sleep technologist must follow. The first step is to determine the patients that require diagnostic testing to confirm the diagnosis of a sleep disorder. This can be achieved through a careful history and physical exam to **establish a baseline** for the patient.

- **History risk factors for sleep disorders:** Snoring while sleeping, witnessed apnea spells, sleep walking, nightmares, excessive movement during sleep, sleepiness during the day, not feeling well rested in the morning, morning headaches, decreased concentration, and psychiatric disorders such as generalized anxiety, depression, and PTSD.

- **Physical exam risk factors for sleep disorders:** Hypertension, obesity, diabetes, congestive heart failure, atrial fibrillation, and the presence of retrognathia (underdeveloped or recessed chin and mandible).

Once a patient at risk for a sleep disorder has been identified, sleep testing can be performed to confirm the diagnosis of a sleep disorder. The severity of the disorder must first be determined before a treatment plan can be put into place. This helps to identify patients at risk for complications. It also helps to formulate an appropriate treatment plan for the patient. The initial assessment information that is gathered in this process will provide a baseline that can be used to assess the effectiveness of the chosen treatment plan.

SUBSTANCE-INDUCED SLEEP DISORDERS

Substance-induced sleep disorder may also result from commonly prescribed drugs.

Drug	Disorder	Characteristics
Antiarrhythmics (quinidine, procainamide)	Insomnia	These drugs may cause disruption of sleep during the night and increased sleepiness in the waking hours.
Antihistamines (diphenhydramine, Benadryl)	Hypersomnia	Some drugs may produce a sedative effect, causing increased sleeping during the night and increased sleepiness during the daytime.
β-Blockers	Insomnia	β-Blockers decrease sleep, increase disruption of sleep, and increase nightmares.
Bronchodilators (theophylline)	Insomnia	High doses of some bronchodilators may cause nervousness, muscle cramping, twitching, and sleep disruption.
Corticosteroids	Insomnia	Steroids may markedly decrease sleep time and increase time needed to fall asleep as well as cause fatigue and jitters during the day.
Diuretics	Insomnia	Decreasing potassium levels may cause leg cramps that interfere with sleeping, and the increase in urinary output may cause nocturia, interrupting sleep.
Nicotine patches	Insomnia	Patches may interfere with falling asleep and duration of sleep and cause vivid dreams or nightmares.
Selective serotonin reuptake inhibitors (SSRIs)	Insomnia	Some individuals experience sleep disruption and sleepiness during waking hours when taking SSRIs.
Thyroid hormone (Synthroid)	Insomnia	High doses of thyroid hormone may cause nervousness, tremors, heart palpitations, and disruption of sleep.

MEDICATIONS THAT CAN CONTRIBUTE TO SLEEP DISORDERS

The following medications may cause or contribute to sleep disorders:

- **Alpha-blockers:** Used to treat hypertension, benign prostatic hyperplasia, and Raynaud's disease. Linked to increased REM sleep and daytime sleepiness.
- **Beta-blockers:** Used to treat hypertension and arrhythmias. May cause nighttime awakenings and nightmares by lowering melatonin levels.
- **Corticosteroids:** Used to treat inflammation and allergic reactions. Can cause insomnia and unpleasant dreams.
- **SSRI antidepressants:** Used to treat depression. Can cause insomnia, mild agitation, and a tremor.
- **ACE inhibitors:** Used to treat hypertension. This class of drugs boosts the body's production of bradykinin, a protein that enlarges blood vessels. This can cause a hacking, dry cough that occurs around the clock and may keep a person awake. It may also cause elevated potassium levels, which can lead to muscle cramps, and can keep a person awake.
- **Angiotensin II-receptor blockers (ARBs):** Used to treat hypertension and heart failure. Like ACE inhibitors, these can cause elevated potassium, which causes muscle cramps.
- **Antihistamines:** Used to treat allergic reactions. May cause anxiety and insomnia in some people.
- **Statins:** Used to treat high cholesterol. May cause insomnia or muscle pain, which can interfere with sleep.

MEDICATIONS THAT MAY INTERFERE WITH SLEEP STUDIES

The following medications can/may interfere with sleep study results:

- **Anti-anxiety medications:** Specifically, benzodiazepines (Ativan, Valium, Xanax) can cause a reduced time of sleep onset and increased total sleep time.
- **Antidepressants:** Tricyclic antidepressants (amitriptyline, nortriptyline) can cause decreased sleep latency and wakefulness. They may also increase limb movements during sleep. Selective serotonin reuptake inhibitors (Prozac, Zoloft) can cause increased limb movements during sleep also, as well as rolling eye movements.
- **Antihypertensives:** The beta-blocker class of medications (atenolol, metoprolol) can alter sleep-waking function. This includes fatigue, insomnia, nightmares, and vivid dreams.
- **Antiseizure medications:** Patients taking these medications (phenobarbital, Dilantin) have increased sleepiness and prolonged sleeping times.
- **Opioids:** These medications (Oxycontin, Vicodin) can cause respiratory depression, which is accentuated in patients with chronic respiratory diseases, and may cause slower ventilations during a sleep study. The symptoms of respiratory depression with these medications may be exaggerated during sleep.

PATIENT ORIENTATION

Patient orientation begins with the patient's arrival at the facility. Orientation should include:

- **Introduction:** The patient should be introduced to the technician and any other staff members who may be present. This is especially important if the patient is to be awakened.
- **Tour of physical plant:** The initial tour should include the patient's individual sleeping area and storage space as well as the bathroom and shower facilities. The patient should observe the technician's monitoring area and any monitoring equipment.

- **Equipment:** The technician should identify and explain the bedside equipment used to monitor sleep.
- **Alarms:** Any alarms or call bells should be demonstrated so the patient knows how to use them and recognizes the sound.
- **Lights/fans:** The patient should know the location of light switches, temperature controls (if available), and fans and should receive instructions on their use.
- **Patient's rights:** The technician should apprise the patient of his or her rights, including the right to privacy and confidentiality and the right to refuse treatment, according to the rules of the Health Insurance Portability and Accountability Act.

PRE-SLEEP INTERVIEW

Pre-sleep interviews are conducted by sleep technicians, who ask questions to clarify information and make careful observations of the patient during the interview, noting the patient's appearance; level of alertness; readiness to learn or obstacles to learning (e.g., language differences, dementia); mental age; and physical limitations, such as hearing impairment or paralysis. The patient's emotional state is assessed as well as any concerns the patient may have about the testing. For example, patients with post-traumatic stress disorder may react violently if awakened abruptly during the night, so the sleep technician must learn about the patient's preferred method of being aroused before testing. Patients with claustrophobia may not be able to tolerate a facemask. The technician notes information gained from the interview on the patient's record. In most sleep centers, a general questionnaire, including a history and a list of medications, is completed before the presleep questionnaire. The general questionnaire is compared with the physician's history and physical, and any additions or discrepancies are noted.

PATIENT IDENTIFICATION AND INFORMED CONSENT

Patients' identification is checked by the sleep technician, following protocol established by the facility, and the records are reviewed carefully to ensure that the correct patient identifier is on all paper and computer records.

Informed consent is provided by patients or family for all treatments the patient receives. This includes a thorough explanation of all procedures and treatments with their associated risks. Patients or family are apprised of all options and allowed input on the types of treatment. Patients or family are apprised of all reasonable risks and any complications that might be life-threatening or increase morbidity. The American Medical Association has established guidelines for informed consent:

- Explanation of diagnosis.
- Nature of, and reason for, treatment or procedure.
- Risks and benefits.
- Alternative options (regardless of cost or insurance coverage).
- Risks and benefits of alternative options.
- Risks and benefits of not having a treatment or procedure.
- Providing informed consent (a requirement of all states)..]

OBTAINING CONSENT FROM PEDIATRIC POPULATION

Informed consent for medical treatments and testing cannot be provided by children younger than 18 years of age (minors), unless they are legally emancipated, until they reach the age of majority, except for certain treatments or testing approved by law, such as for birth control, abortion, and HIV testing; however, even laws concerning these situations vary from state to state, with some requiring parental notification. However, children must be included in discussions about treatment options and testing in accordance with their age and level of understanding. Because children do not always appreciate cause and effect relationships, the law allows the parents to override decisions of the child and teenager, but forcing a child to have treatment or testing puts the child in a poor emotional state and is cause for ethical concern. Therefore, the sleep technician should work with both the parents and the child, explaining the benefits and disadvantages of testing, to bring about agreement or assent on the part of the child. This is especially important for adolescents, who are seeking autonomy.

HIPAA

HIPAA regulations are designed to protect the rights of individuals regarding the privacy of their health information. The technician must not release any information or documentation about a patient's condition or treatment without consent, as the individual has the right to determine who has access to personal information. Personal information about the patient is considered protected health information and consists of any identifying or personal information about the patient, such as health history, condition, treatments in any form, and any documentation, including electronic, verbal, or written. Personal information can be shared with parents of minors, spouses, legal guardians, those with durable power of attorney for the patient, and those involved in the care of the patient, such as physicians, without a specific release, but the patient should always be consulted if personal information is to be discussed with others present to ensure there is no objection. Failure to comply with HIPAA regulations can make a technician liable for legal action.

CONFIDENTIALITY

Confidentiality is the obligation that is present in a professional-patient relationship. technicians are under an obligation to protect the information they possess concerning the patient and family. Care should be taken to safeguard that information and provide the privacy that the family deserves. This is accomplished through the use of required passwords when the family calls for information about the patient and through the limitations of who is allowed to visit There may be times when confidentiality must be broken to save the life of a patient, but those circumstances are rare. The technician must make all efforts to safeguard patient records and identification. Computerized record-keeping should be done in such a way that the screen is not visible to others, and paper records must be secured.

> **Review Video: Ethics and Confidentiality in Counseling**
> Visit mometrix.com/academy and enter code: 250384

PATIENTS' RIGHTS

Patients' (families') rights concerning what to expect from a health care organization are outlined in the standards of both the Joint Commission and the National Committee for Quality Assurance. Rights include:

- Respect for the patient, including personal dignity and psychosocial, spiritual, and cultural considerations.
- Response to needs related to access and pain control.
- Ability to make decisions about care, including informed consent, advance directives, and end-of-life care.
- Procedure for registering complaints or grievances.
- Protection of confidentiality and privacy.
- Freedom from abuse or neglect.
- Protection during research and information related to ethical issues of research.

20

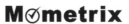

- Appraisal of outcomes, including unexpected outcomes.
- Information about organization, services, and practitioners.
- Appeal procedures for decisions regarding benefits and quality of care.
- Organizational code of ethical behavior.
- Procedures for donating and procuring organs and tissue.

SLEEP DIARIES

Sleep diaries are invaluable to the patients' assessment. The patient keeps a record of sleep habits for a 2-week period preceding the test. The sleep diary generally has two components:

- **Before sleep:** Patient assesses mood with a 1-5 scale that ranges from bad mood to excellent mood, notes any medications taken (especially sleeping medications) and the time the lights are turned off.
- **Upon awakening:** Patient estimates the approximate time to onset of sleep and the number of arousals during the night and the time of awakening. The patient assesses mood with a 1-5 scale.

Patient's perceptions about the time needed to fall asleep and the number of awakenings that occur during the night may be considerably at odds with the findings during the polysomnogram. The patient may simply be mistaken, or the patient's experience in the sleep center is different. For example, some people find it very difficult to sleep during the test or may arouse more easily in a strange environment.

PRE-SLEEP QUESTIONNAIRE

Pre-sleep questionnaires are usually standardized forms that review issues related to sleep, but the technician asks additional questions for clarification as needed. The questionnaire helps to determine if the patient's preceding 24 hours were normal for that individual. Topics covered include the following:

Sleep preparation	Activities done before bedtime, such as showering, exercising, watching television, or reading in bed
Sleep patterns	Usual time to bed, time to rise, and time needed to fall asleep
Sleep position	Side lying, supine, prone, and number of pillows
Sleep problems	Restlessness, restless legs, insomnia, snoring, gasping, choking, or apneic periods
Sleep arrangement	Sleeps alone, has bed partner, or sleeps with animals on bed
Sleep aids	Sleeping medications, music, television, or reading
Habits	Smoking, drinking, including the type, amount, and time used within 24 hours of testing
Nocturia	Frequency of using the bathroom during the night
Other physical complaints	Dry mouth on arising, nasal congestion, or headaches in the morning
Daytime patterns	Sleepiness in the morning, tiredness through day, falling asleep inappropriately, needing naps, and duration and frequency of naps
Medications	All medications taken within 24 hours of testing

BED-PARTNER QUESTIONNAIRES

Bed-partner questionnaires are filled out by the patient's bed partner (or in some cases a roommate or parent) with the patient's permission. The partner is often aware of snoring or periods of apnea, even though the patient may not be aware. A typical questionnaire includes the following information:

- Patient and reporter's names.
- Frequency with which the reporter has observed the patient sleeping.
- Positions in which the patient typically sleeps (back, stomach, right side, left side) and an estimate of the percentage of the night in each position.
- Descriptions of sleep behaviors (usually with a checklist):
  o Type of snoring: light, loud, or snorting.
  o Respiratory changes: choking or pauses.
  o Extremities: twitching or jerking.
  o Seizure-like activity: rigidity or shaking.
  o Mouth activity: teeth grinding.
  o Abnormal sleep behavior: sleep walking, talking, crying, sitting up, banging head, or rocking.
  o Awakening behavior: alert, lethargic, or complaining of pain.

MORNING/EVENING QUESTIONNAIRES

Morning/Evening questionnaires ask nineteen questions about time preferences, providing a range of answers that determines if the person is a morning, evening, or neutral person. (In 1976, Horne and Ostberg studied sleep patterns and classified people as "morning" or "evening" people, depending on their preferences for sleeping and arising and level of alertness.) Questions include:

- The time of day the patient would get up and go to bed if free to decide; The degree of dependency on an alarm clock to awaken at the normally scheduled time; The ease of getting up in the morning
- The patient's feelings and appetite in the half hour after awakening
- The time of day the patient gets up on days with no obligations in relation to normal time to arise; The ease with which the patient could engage in sports activities between 7 and 8 am or 10 and 11 pm; The time of day at which the patient feels tired enough to fall asleep; The 2 hours during the day the patient would prefer to study for an exam; How the patient feels in the morning after going to sleep at 11 pm; The time the patient would arise after going to bed several hours late; when the patient would sleep if having to stand guard from 4-6 am; The 2 hours during the day the patient would prefer to exercise; The 5 consecutive hours during the day the patient would prefer to work; The hour the patient feels the best; Whether the patient considers him- or herself a morning or evening person.

Technical Preparation

PATIENT ROOMS

Patient rooms vary considerably but should be as non-institution-like as possible with at least 140 square feet recommended for each patient. The bed should be positioned so that staff can access the patient on both sides. Adjustable beds provide more comfort to help patients relax. Blackout blinds should be available to block outside lights at night and ambient daylight for daytime napping. When possible, the day and nighttime room temperatures should be set to the patient's preference. Fans

22

or extra blankets should be available if individual room temperatures cannot be set. Restrooms should be clean and easily available to the patient. Shared bathrooms must be monitored and cleaned frequently. Storage space should be adequate to contain patient's clothing and toiletries as well as equipment and supplies needed during testing. If showers are available for patient use, they should be stocked with individual soap, shampoo, and towels.

EQUIPMENT INSPECTION

Inspection of equipment should precede the examination. Before beginning the polysomnogram, the equipment is thoroughly inspected to ensure that the system is connected to electricity, that all cables and wires are secure, and that the equipment is functioning properly. The computer is turned on, and the patient information file is opened to ensure that information about the patient was entered correctly into the system. Any equipment issues, such as malfunctioning or incompatibility, are resolved before beginning the test as this may impact the results. All necessary supplies and equipment, such as leads, glue, and tape, are laid out and easily accessible to avoid unnecessary delays, thereby reducing patient stress. The physician's orders should be checked to verify that the correct montage has been selected.

ELECTROENCEPHALOGRAMS

Electroencephalograms (EEGs) measure the electrical activity within the brain through scalp electrodes to rule out seizure disorders and to determine the characteristics of the sleep-wake state. Waves/cycles in 1 second are measured in Hertz (Hz) to determine the stage of sleep:

$$\text{Alpha} = 8 - 13 \text{ Hz}$$
$$\text{Beta} = 13 - 30 \text{ Hz}$$
$$\text{Delta} =< 0.5 - 4 \text{ Hz}$$
$$\text{Theta} => 4 - 7 \text{ Hz}$$

The EEG equipment may be analog, with waves recorded on paper, or digital, with waves recorded electronically for viewing on a computer screen. All equipment should be properly calibrated, and paper should be inserted before use (for analog). Digital EEG equipment is usually used instead of analog because it presents a more accurate reading and allows a variety of filters for different montages. The EEG can be set to display the electroencephalograph in page mode (usually showing 10-second increments) or in continuous scroll mode. Typically, six leads are used (including two reference leads) although more may be applied to diagnose seizure disorders.

ELECTROCARDIOGRAMS

Electrocardiograms (ECGs) record and show a graphic display of the electrical activity of the heart through a number of different waveforms, complexes, and intervals:

- **P wave:** The P wave represents the beginning of electrical impulses in the sinus node, which spread through the atria (muscle depolarization).
- **QRS complex:** The QRS complex represents ventricular muscle depolarization and atrial repolarization.
- **T wave:** The T wave represents ventricular muscle repolarization (resting state) as cells regain negative charge.
- **U wave:** The U wave represents repolarization of the Purkinje fibers.

A modified lead II ECG is typically used for polysomnography to identify basic heart rhythms and dysrhythmias. Typical placement of leads for a 2-lead ECG is 3-5 cm inferior to the right clavicle and left lower ribcage. Typical placement for a 3-lead ECG is the right arm near the shoulder (RA), V_5 position over the 5th intercostal space (LA), and the left upper leg near the groin (LL).

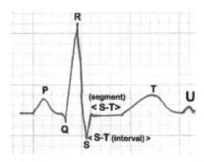

ANTERIOR TIBIALIS ELECTROMYOGRAMS

Anterior tibialis electromyograms (atEMGs) monitor the electrical activity in the leg muscles, allowing for monitoring of periodic leg movement during the polysomnogram because electrical activity is absent when the muscle is relaxed and increases with movement. The atEMG may show twitching and slight muscle activity and movement that may not be obvious by observation alone. Typically, muscle activity slows during sleep, especially during stage R sleep, so that people are not active while dreaming. While intramuscular leads are used to diagnose neuromuscular disorders, surface leads are used for polysomnography because only a general overview of muscle activity is needed. In some cases, if respiratory effort is being monitored, leads may be placed intercostally.

USE OF PULSE OXIMETRY DURING A PSG

Pulse oximetry, continuous or intermittent, uses an external oximeter that attaches to the patient's finger (or earlobe) to measure arterial oxygen saturation (SpO_2), the percentage of hemoglobin that is saturated with oxygen. The oximeter also indicates the current heart rate. The oximeter uses light waves to determine SpO_2. Normal SpO_2 should be over 95% although some patients with chronic respiratory disorders, such as chronic obstructive pulmonary disease may have lower SpO_2 values. Impaired circulation, excessive light, poor positioning, and nail polish may compromise results. If SpO_2 falls, the oximeter should be repositioned, as an incorrect position is a common cause of inaccurate readings. Oximeters do not provide information about carbon dioxide levels, so they cannot monitor carbon dioxide retention. The oximeter is usually placed on an index finger but may be placed on an earlobe if necessary.

RECORDED ELECTRICAL ACTIVITY

Electrical activity is recorded by the polysomnogram (PSG) as tracings from three signal sources.

- **Bioelectrical signals:** These are generated by the patient's tissue and motion and recorded by surface electrodes to the display of the electroencephalogram, electrocardiogram, electrooculogram, and electromyogram.
- **Transduced signals:** These derive from sensors that convert action, such as chest wall movement, into electrical signals with the electrical signal generated by the sensor instead of the body.
- **Equipment signals:** Sometimes ancillary equipment, such as a carbon dioxide analyzer, is used during the PSG. This equipment, which has separate signal displays, outputs, and processing units, may be stand-alone or interfaced with the digital PSG equipment.

FACE ELECTRODES

Face electrodes are used to ground and to record eye and chin activity and include:

- **Ground electrode:** This electrode does not impact measurements with modern computerized equipment. It is usually placed in the middle of the forehead but can be placed anywhere on the body.
- **Electrooculogram (EOG):** The EOG records vertical and horizontal eye movements and helps to identify periods of REM sleep. Pairs of electrodes are placed with one pair by the right eye and the other by the left.
- **Chin electromyogram (cEMG):** The cEMG records muscle tone of the chin muscles and helps to identify REM sleep, during which muscle tone decreases. The cEMG can also provide information about teeth grinding, which causes muscle movement, and snoring, as snoring causes artifacts.

PURPOSE OF SENSORS DURING A PSG

Sensors may be used during the polysomnogram to provide additional information about breathing during sleep:

- **Respiratory effort:** Piezo-sensor bands or respiratory inductive plethysmography are used to indicate chest and abdominal movement during respiration as an indirect means of representing respiratory effort.
- **Snore:** Microphones or piezo-sensors applied to the lateral-anterior neck superior to the larynx are used to indicate the degree and duration of snoring. Sensors are more accurate than microphones.
- **Airflow:** Thermal sensors (thermistors or thermocouples) or pressure transducers (nasal) monitor both intake and outflow of air through the nostrils and the mouth. Typically, two prongs are inserted into the nose and a third prong is in front of the mouth.

APPLICATION OF EEG ELECTRODES AND SENSORS

Electroencephalogram (EEG) electrodes and sensors must be applied properly in the correct position. EEG electrodes are placed using the international 10/20 measuring system, which uses the nasion, inion, and preauricular points as landmarks while measuring the skull to determine lead placement at 10%-20% distance from the landmarks. EEG leads are designated, according to the part of the skull to which they are applied, with even numbered subscripts on the right and odd numbered subscripts on the left. The system reference electrode is placed according to software requirements, often the central lead (C_z) at the vertex or top center of the head. Sleep technology often requires only a modified EEG with fewer electrodes, typically right and left central (C_4 and C_3), right and left occipital (O_2 and O_1), and right and left reference mastoid leads (A_2 and A_1).

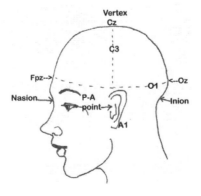

C$_z$ Scalp Electrode Site

Scalp electrode site measuring uses the international 10/20 measuring system based on landmarks (e.g., nasion, inion, preauricular points). Sleep technicians must be proficient at performing these site measurements. Points are labeled, according to area of the brain and the exact site, so O$_1$ is occipital area 1 with odd numbers indicating the left side:

C$_z$ is measured vertically from the inion to the nasion and midline. The technician marks the 50% (vertex) measure at the top of the head as well as a 10% and two 20% measures on each side of the vertex, starting at the nasion and inion. The technician then measures from the left preauricular point to the right, intersecting at the 50% mark (vertex) and marking a 10% and two 20% measures on each side of the vertex, starting at the preauricular points. The point where the two vertical lines intersect at the vertex is C$_z$.

Additional Scalp Electrode Sites

Other scalp electrode sites are measured once the vertical lines connecting the nasion and inion and the preauricular points are drawn and C$_z$ is identified. The technician measures the following:

- **F$_{pz}$ and O$_z$:** A vertical line is drawn 10% superior to the nasion, midline, to identify F$_{pz}$ and 10% superior to the inion to identify O$_z$. A horizontal line is drawn 10% above the preauricular points to create a horizontal line that circles the head through O$_z$ and F$_{pz}$.
- **C$_3$:** On the 30% mark (10% plus 20%) above the left preauricular point.
- **C$_4$:** On the 30% mark (10% plus 20%) above the right preauricular point.
- **O$_1$:** On the 5% mark to the left of O$_z$ on the horizontal line that is 10% above the left preauricular point.
- **O$_2$:** On the 5% mark to the right of O$_z$ on the horizontal line that is 10% above the right preauricular point.
- **A$_1$:** Over the left mastoid process behind ear.
- **A$_2$:** Over the right mastoid process behind ear.

Face, Electrooculogram, and Chin Electromyogram Electrode Placement

Face, electrooculogram (EOG), and chin electromyogram (cEMG) electrode placement during polysomnography include the following:

Ground electrode	Place electrode on central forehead on line between nasion and hairline on a flat area of skin, avoiding deep wrinkles or creases.
EOG	Right electrode: Place electrode 1 cm lateral to and 1 cm superior to the outer canthus.
	Left electrode: Place electrode 1 cm lateral to and 1 cm inferior to the outer canthus.
cEMG	Method 1: Place two electrodes on chin, 3 cm apart and 2 cm below lower lip.
	Method 2: Place two electrodes on submentalis muscle, 3 cm apart (advised for thin but not obese patients).
	Method 3: Place one electrode on the chin (center) and the other on the submentalis muscle.
Anterior tibialis electromyogram	Place two electrodes 3 cm apart along the anterior tibialis ridges on both legs, avoiding the tibias.

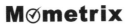

SENSORS FOR RESPIRATORY EFFORT, SNORE, AIRFLOW, AND OXIMETER

Sensors, such as respiratory effort, snore, airflow, and oximeter, are used during polysomnography.

Respiratory effort	Bands (sized for the individual patient) containing sensors are placed securely (being careful not to restrict breathing) about the patient's body with lead wires pointed upwards: Thorax: Secured just below axilla. Abdomen: Secured about the waist.
Snore	Microphone: Placed close to the patient.
	Sensor: Placed laterally on the anterior neck, superior to the larynx.
Airflow	Nasal prongs are inserted into the nostrils, and the third prong is positioned in front of the mouth.
Oximeter	The oximeter is clipped to the index finger closest to oximeter or to the earlobe.

HEAD AND FACE ELECTRODE SITES AND ATTACHMENT METHODS

Head and face electrodes are applied to areas that are clean and free of oil to ensure good quality signals. Before attachment, the skin must be cleaned thoroughly with an alcohol swab and then scrubbed for 5-10 seconds with an abrasive skin cleanser, such as NuPrep, using a cotton swab and being sure to scrub only the area of attachment, carefully separating the hair on the scalp.

COLLODION ATTACHMENT

Collodion attachment involves placing the electrode on the scrubbed site and covered with 2-3-cm size square of single-ply gauze. The air compressor stylus is inserted through the gauze and into the top center of the electrode and then collodion glue is applied with an eyedropper to saturate the gauze. Smooth gauze is placed over the scalp or skin while drying with an air compressor, using care to avoid getting glue between the electrode and the skin. The stylus is removed. Using a blunt-tipped needle, the electrode is filled with electrolyte gel/cream.

ELECTRODE CREAM AND TAPE ATTACHMENT

Head and face electrodes are applied by different methods after the skin is scrubbed, including:

- **Electrode cream attachment:** Electrode cream (EC2), which is an adhesive, is applied to one side of a 3-cm square of single-ply gauze. The electrode cup is filled with electrolyte paste/conductive gel, and the lead is placed in the middle of the gauze (gel side facing upward) to secure it to the gauze; the electrode and the gauze are then inverted onto the scrubbed skin, smoothing the gauze over the skin to secure it.
- **Electrode tape attachment (electrode collar):** The electrode cup is filled with electrolyte paste/conductive gel and inverted onto the skin. The electrode is covered with tape, which is smoothed to secure it to the skin. The electrode is tucked under a corner of the tape to facilitate later removal.

Electrode leads from the face and scalp should be gathered together and secured with tape or Velcro every 4-6 inches to prevent tangling.

APPLICATION OF BODY ELECTRODES

Body electrode sites include those for the electrocardiogram (ECG) and the anterior tibialis electromyogram (atEMG). Applying the electrodes includes:

- **Skin preparation:** Electrode placement sites are thoroughly cleaned with alcohol, using a cotton applicator or premoistened alcohol swab. An abrasive cleaner, such as NuPrep, is indicated only if impedance is high. If the patient is hairy (primarily men), the area may need to be shaved before cleaning the skin.
- **Application:**
  - **ECG:** The lead wire is attached to the electrode before application. The adhesive backing is removed, and the gel side is placed against the skin, feeding the wires through the patient's clothing, and then plugging them into the appropriate jack.
  - **atEMG:** Electrodes are attached with a double-sided electrode collar and taped (2 inches). The electrode wires are looped between the electrodes and secured to prevent dislodgment during the exam.

VERIFYING IMPEDANCES

Verifying impedances is done by the technician after calibrating the machine to determine if the electrodes are properly applied and signal quality is appropriate. Electrodes pick up the electrical current generated by tissue and transmit this signal to the machine, which creates a wave pattern. If the connection between the electrode and the conducting gel is disrupted, the signal is distorted, causing motion artifacts. Silver/silver chloride electrodes tend to have less motion artifacts than gold electrodes. Impedance refers to interference with the electrical signal from the point of contact to the recording device. Each type of electrode has an associated source impedance, but impedance levels for each individual electrode should remain low (≤ 5 kilohms). Each electrode should be individually tested, using the internal impedance meter or an external handheld meter. A difference in impedance between paired electrodes increases artifacts. If the impedance level of an electrode is high, then the electrode may need to be repositioned.

WRIST ACTIGRAPHY

Wrist actigraphy uses a portable device worn on the wrist that records and analyzes movement. Information stored in the device is downloaded into a computer. A number of different devices are available, and they evaluate movement in different ways, using a single channel, so determining the validity of the reports or comparing it to standard polysomnography is problematic, especially if patients have movement disorders or periods of quiet (without moving) during waking hours. Because of these limitations, wrist actigraphy should be used for multiple days (at least three 24-hour periods with up to 7 days optimal) to help to identify patterns of sleep/waking. Wrist actigraphy alone is not usually adequate for diagnosis of sleep disordered breathing or periodic limb movement but can be used to evaluate other sleep disorders. The patient should keep a diary of activities during wrist actigraphy to identify artifacts and to aid in interpretation of the results. Scoring varies, according to the manufacturer's guidelines.

MONTAGE SELECTION

Selection of the montage depends on the presumptive diagnosis and the type of testing.

Nocturnal polysomnogram (PSG)	EEG, EOG, cEMG, atEMG, pulse oximetry, and sensors for respiratory effort, snore, and airflow.	Used to diagnose obstructive sleep apnea syndrome and may be done before MSLT.

Multiple sleep latency test (MSLT)	EEG (central and occipital), EOG cEMG, and ECG; other channels are optional.	Used to diagnose excessive sleepiness (hypersomnia) and narcolepsy during waking hours; done after nocturnal PSG to ensure 6 hours of sleep preceding test.
Maintenance of wakefulness test	Same as for MSLT.	Used to evaluate success of treatment or ability to stay awake during the daytime; does not usually require a nocturnal PSG although it may be indicated for shift workers.

CHILDREN WITH NEUROMUSCULAR DISEASES

Montage requirements for children with neuromuscular diseases are listed below.

EEG, EOG, and cEMG	Sleep staging shows progression of disease.
	Mild: Frequent arousal and decreased stage R sleep and stage N1 sleep
	Moderate: Frequent arousals and awakening and deceased stage R sleep
	Advanced: Short arousal and awakening after prolonged periods of desaturation and absent stage R sleep.
Oximetry	Mild: ≤ 96%
	Moderate: ≤ 94% with desaturation during stage R sleep
	Advanced: ≤ 92% with desaturation during all sleep stages
Respiratory effort	Respiratory effort varies with the type of disorder and the degree of muscle impairment; thus, it may be difficult to judge respiratory effort. Inductance plethysmography is most accurate.
Airflow	Mild: Respiratory rate is increased.
	Moderate: Respiratory rate is normal to increased.
	Advanced: Respiratory rate is normal.
	Snoring may indicate obstruction.
etCO$_2$ continue transition monitoring.	Mild: < 45 torr
	Moderate: ≥ 45 torr
	Advanced: ≥ 50 torr
	Increases may be evident before oxygen desaturation with onset of hypoventilation.
ECG	Cardiac arrhythmias are common with neuromuscular diseases.
Video	Correlating activity with recordings is essential.

Abbreviations: EEG = electroencephalogram; EOG = electrooculogram; cEMG = chin electromyogram; ECG = electrocardiogram; and etCO$_2$ = end-tidal carbon dioxide.

NONINVASIVE VENTILATION

Noninvasive ventilation (NIV) is used with patients with neuromuscular disease to prevent or delay respiratory failure and the use of more invasive ventilatory measures; however, in some cases, such as Duchenne's muscular dystrophy, too early use of NIV may worsen respiratory failure. NIV may be implemented during polysomnography. Factors to consider include:

- Gas exchange goals: This includes acceptable oxygen saturation and carbon dioxide levels and parameters for use. The physician's orders should explicitly state the levels at which NIV is to be implemented.
- Type of ventilation, device, and settings.
- Accessibility of a physician in case of emergencies.
- Interface: The oronasal mask must be used with care for neuromuscular patients because they cannot easily remove the mask. Nasal prongs may not be an appropriate fit for small children and may not provide adequate ventilation.

EQUIPMENT CALIBRATION

Equipment calibration (with standard settings for filters and sensitivity) of 30 seconds must be done and recorded before beginning the polysomnogram after the leads and sensors are applied and the patient is quiet. Calibration procedures vary somewhat, depending on the software and equipment used, so manufacturer's instructions should be noted and followed. Electroencephalograms, electrooculograms, and electromyograms generally require negative 50 microvolts per centimeter DC to all channels to obtain a deflection of the recording pen in the range of 5-10 mm. The technician visually examines each calibration wave. As part of the calibration procedure, the technician makes sure the equipment is properly plugged in, that all jacks are placed correctly, and that signal quality is adequate. Leads and sensors should be adjusted to control impedances and artifacts. Upon completion of the study, usually within 8 hours, the calibration procedure is repeated for 30 seconds, and results are compared with the initial calibration to ensure accuracy during the recording period.

PHYSIOLOGICAL (BIO-) CALIBRATIONS

Physiological (bio-) calibrations are performed by the technician to evaluate signals generated by the patient:

- **Electrocardiogram (ECG):** The technician checks the polarity of the reading to ensure the ECG tracing is not inverted, which is a sign that the jacks are inserted in incorrect channels.
- **Electroencephalogram (EEG):** The technician asks the patient to relax with the eyes open for 30 seconds or more, during which time the alpha waves on the EEG are typically prominent. Then the patient is asked to close the eyes for 30 seconds.
- **Electrooculogram (EOG):** When the patient is relaxed with the head still, the technician asks the patient to look to the right and to the left a number of times, up and down a number of times, and finally to blink slowly about 5 times; the technician then examines the EOG tracings to ensure that the three different types of eye movements are distinct on the recording.

Physiological (bio-) calibrations that must be completed before the polysomnogram (PSG) include:

- **Chin electromyogram (cEMG):** The technician asks the patient to relax and remain quiet while determining that baseline muscle tone remains at 5 cm/amplitude or more. Then, the patient is asked to swallow, grit the teeth, and bite down to ensure that these actions show activity on the cEMG recording.

- **Anterior tibialis electromyogram (atEMG):** The technician asks the patient to extend the legs and then to flex and extend the great toe on each foot, which should show activity on the atEMG tracings.
- **Snore sensor:** The technician asks the patient to count to five out loud as this should cause deflection.
- **Respiratory effort sensors and airflow sensors:** The technician asks the patient to stop breathing and hold the breath in briefly to ensure that the respiratory tracing shows a flat line. The patient is then asked to mimic paradoxical breathing by tightening and relaxing the thorax.

Physiological calibrations should be repeated at the end of the PSG to ensure that leads and sensors remain in the correct position and that recordings were accurate.

SAMPLING RATES

Sampling rates must be selected before testing when converting analog recordings to digital as they cannot be changed afterward in the way that filters can be changed. The converter uses predetermined intervals to assign a numeric value to waveforms. This value determines the amplitude (height) of the waveform. The sampling rate is equal to the number of sampled intervals done in 1 second. According to sampling theory, the minimum sampling rate is equal to at least twice the highest frequency sampled, but this will not provide an accurate representation of the analog waveform, so a higher sampling rate is necessary to achieve an adequate waveform. For example, sampling rates must be about 10 times higher for electroencephalograms (200-300 Hz with 30-35 Hz high-frequency settings) with adjustments if high-frequency filter settings are increased. Sampling rates should be selected for each channel.

PURPOSE OF FILTERS

Filters are used to gain a more accurate recording by isolating bandwidths and reducing outside interference, such as from signals produced by the skin or muscle activity that causes artifacts. Most digital equipment records without the use of filters, but filters can later be applied to "clean up" the recording; however, filters (especially low frequency) can cause a phase shift that causes the wave to appear earlier or later. Filters are set in relation to the normal bandwidth of the test.

- **Low-frequency filters** eliminate signals below the normal bandwidth for a particular test.
- **High-frequency filters** eliminate signals above the normal bandwidth for a particular test.
- **60 Hz notch (band reject) filters** remove signals (noise) produced in the 50-60 Hz range (power line interference) without affecting other frequencies, but this filter can interfere with recordings so it is rarely used except for anterior tibialis electromyograms.
- **Band-pass filters** record frequencies only within a particular range.

FREQUENCY SETTING OPTIONS FOR FILTERS

Frequency settings for filters vary, according to the test.

- **Electroencephalogram (EEG) [standard sensitivity of 50 microvolts/cm]:** Usually recorded in the range of 0.5-25 Hz, a low-frequency filter, therefore, would be set below the bottom range (at about 0.3), effectively reducing output below that level, and a high-frequency filter would be set above the top range (at 30-35 Hz), although when used to diagnose seizure activity, the high-frequency filter needs to be set higher (70-75 Hz) to allow for spiking during epileptic activity. Time constant is 0.25 seconds.
- **Electrooculogram:** Settings are similar to those for an EEG.

- **Chin electromyogram (cEMG) and EMG:** The low-frequency filters are typically set at 10 Hz, and the high-frequency filters are set at 90-100 Hz. Time constant is 0.1 seconds.
- **Electrocardiogram (sensitivity at 1 millivolt/cm):** The low-frequency filter is set at 1 Hz, and the high-frequency filters are set at 30-35 Hz. Time constant is 0.1 seconds.
- **Respiratory sensors:** The low-frequency filters are set at 0.1 Hz, and the high-frequency filters are set at 0.5 Hz. Time constant is 1 second.
- **Oximetry (sensitivity at 1 volt/cm):** The high-frequency filter is set at 15 Hz.

IMPACT OF FILTERS ON APPEARANCE OF WAVEFORM

The appearance of the waveform is affected by filters. During calibration, when a 50-microvolt negative DC voltage is applied without filters, the waveform takes on a square appearance with an upward spike that is then sustained for the duration the voltage is applied. With low- and high-frequency filter settings, the shape and duration of waveforms alter as do the time constants, the difference between constant rise time and constant fall time:

- **Rise time:** Interval of time required for calibration waves to rise to 63% of amplitude.
- **Fall time:** Interval of time required for calibration waves to fall to 37% of amplitude.

Changing the setting of high- and low-frequency filters directly affects rise and fall time. Lowering the high-frequency filter setting increases rise time. Lowering the low-frequency filter setting increases fall time.

FREQUENCY AND AMPLITUDE

Frequency and amplitude are waveforms that are recorded on polysomnography, using a standard time scale of 1 cm/sec. Frequency is the number of waves/cycles generated per second, and amplitude is the vertical height of a wave, determined by electrical voltage.

Machines are calibrated with a known signal so that waveforms can be interpreted according to height and sensitivity settings. The setting of 50 microvolts/cm, typically used for electroencephalo-grams, electrooculograms, chin electromyograms, and electromyograms, means that 50 microvolts of signal produce a standardized waveform that is 1 cm high. The wave height varies in relation to the sensitivity setting. While digital machines can record in a variety of ways, the data are displayed and recorded so that frequency and amplitude can be visually confirmed.

Procedures and Protocols

BASIC PROTOCOLS FOR ADULT PSG STUDIES

Ideally, the patient's medical chart should be reviewed before they arrive for the sleep study to review any pertinent medical history. Before beginning the study, the patient's identity should be confirmed, vital signs should be taken, and a review of any medications taken in the past 24 hours. Before applying the electrodes, the skin should be cleaned to ensure adequate conduction of signals. This includes leads for EKG, EEG, EMG, and EOG. The pulse oximeter clip should be placed on a finger. A thoracic band may be applied to record any thoracic or abdominal movement. Electrodes are placed on the arms and legs, also, to measure any limb movements. A nasal cannula is placed to measure air pressure during sleep. Electrodes are placed over the diaphragm to record EMG measurements of the diaphragm. A microphone is also placed to record snoring. Before beginning the study, a test should be done to ensure all of the electrodes are recording information accurately. The video recorder should also be tested to ensure the entire patient is visible.

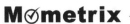

MODIFICATIONS FOR INFANT POLYSOMNOGRAMS

Infant polysomnograms (PSGs) may be done for short (between feedings) or extended (overnight) periods, but short examinations may not render adequate information, so longer testing is recommended. Some modifications are necessary for infant PSGs. Usually a parent or caregiver remains in the room with the infant although the person should be advised not to disturb the child except for feeding and diaper changes during the test. For toddlers, the room should be as child friendly as possible. The temperature is usually maintained at about 23°C, and the child should be in a crib or secure bed with side rails. Using play and dolls to show placement of electrodes may be helpful for small children. Safety measures should be in place to secure all electrical outlets, supplies, and equipment.

PLACEMENT OF SENSORS AND OXIMETER FOR INFANT POLYSOMNOGRAMS

Sensors for the infant polysomnogram must be placed carefully to ensure accurate recording.

- **Respiratory effort sensors:** It is important that the sensors (inductance plethysmography or piezo crystal bands) are the correct size and secured with tape if necessary. The thoracic band is placed immediately above the nipple and the abdominal band, about the umbilicus.
- **Position sensor:** This sensor is placed according to the manufacturer's directions, usually on the lower back (over the diaper) with the infant in the supine position.
- **Motion sensor:** This sensor is placed on a limb, which is moved to ensure that the signal is adequate.

The oximeter is placed carefully on the hand or foot of the infant, and secured with wrapping as necessary, avoiding excess padding that might increase heat and affect readings.

MODIFICATIONS FOR PLACING ELECTRODES AND SENSORS FOR INFANT/CHILD POLYSOMNOGRAMS

Infant/child polysomnograms (PSGs) may require some modification when placing electrodes and sensors. Parents may hold or soothe the child when leads are applied. There are a number of factors to consider:

- Collodion may cause eye irritation, so paste or another adhesive may be used. Pasted electrodes increase slow-frequency electroencephalogram (EEG) artifacts, reduced by increasing a low-frequency filter to 1 Hz (but this will interfere with slow-wave EEG activity).
- Toddlers may require a gauze turban or cap to keep scalp electrodes in place.
- Infants may need their hands covered with socks, and toddlers may need parents to prevent the child from touching leads until the child is asleep.
- Bundling and taping of leads can prevent dislodgement.
- Re-referencing/re-montaging may be necessary if children are active.
- Higher sampling rates are needed to detect seizure activity (EEG ≥ 500 Hz and electrooculogram/electromyogram ≥ 200 Hz).
- A chin electromyogram should be placed where it will not come in contact with drool.
- Respiratory effort belts and sensors may need to be secured with tape.

pH Sensor in Infant Polysomnograms

A pH sensor may be placed in the esophagus to diagnose gastric acid reflux in infants and children. In infants, a thin wire with a sensor at the end is passed nasally, but older children (or adults) may be able to swallow the sensor with fluids. There are two types of sensors that are used:

- **Antimony/antimony oxide electrode:** The small pellet-like sensor is antimony coated with antimony oxide. A skin reference electrode is needed for this type.
- **Glass electrode:** The glass electrode is a combined sensor and reference electrode (2-4 mm diameter). It is inserted into the esophagus in the same manner as the antimony/antimony oxide electrode. The glass electrode has a high level of electrical impedance that can interfere with readings and can be broken if not handled properly, although it is unlikely to break when positioned in the esophagus.

Interventions During Infant Polysomnogram

Interventions during an infant polysomnogram are made as indicated by what the technologist observes. Emergency action may be needed if an infant has apneic periods for over 20 seconds. The oxygen saturation and heart rate are noted to determine if the infant is showing a decrease, but no intervention is necessary until the oxygen saturation level is less than 85% or the heart rate is less than 60 bpm for 10 seconds. When oxygen saturation and heart rate have fallen to the critical points, intervention is indicated:

- The infant is stimulated by flicking the thumb against the heels or the bottom of the feet.
- If there is no improvement, the airway and position are checked, using suction to clear airways if necessary. Oxygen per bag is provided; a few puffs are administered and continued until oxygen saturation and heart rate return to normal.
- If the infant's condition still does not improve, emergency procedures are followed (a code is called for a physician).
- The electroencephalogram is checked for indications of seizure activity.

Patient Needs Based on Age for Infant/Child Polysomnography

During **infant/child polysomnography**, close observation of children is necessary to relate activities to recorded data, as this information may be critical in developing a diagnosis for sleep-related disorders.

Newborn to 5 years	The lab tries to emulate the sleep environment and activities of the child's home as much as possible, and the technician observes the behaviors of both the child and parents, including interactions and bedtime rituals.
5-12 years	The technician reviews the child's sleep log or parental report of the child's sleeping habits and carefully notes behaviors, such as stalling or tantrums that may delay bedtime. The child's ability to initiate sleep should be observed as well as episodes of fidgeting, restlessness, or crying. Bedtime habits or rituals (e.g., reading, watching television, co-sleeping) are followed and documented as they may affect sleep onset.
12-18 years	While observations are similar to those of adults, adolescents often are concerned about privacy and may feel uncomfortable sleeping under the observation of a technician of the opposite gender; thus, a frank discussion that allows the adolescent to express opinions is important.

AAP Clinical Guidelines for Diagnosis and Treatment of OSAS

The American Academy of Pediatrics has issued clinical guidelines for the diagnosis and treatment of obstructive sleep apnea syndrome (OSAS). Recommendations include:

- All children are screened for snoring, observed apnea, restlessness during sleep, daytime sleepiness, or neurobehavioral abnormalities.
- Physical exam notes abnormalities that may relate to OSAS.
- If indications of OSAS are present:
  - High-risk children with co-morbid conditions should be immediately referred to a specialist.
  - Children who are not high risk but show evidence of cardiac or respiratory failure should have further evaluation in consultation with a specialist.
  - Children who are not high risk and do not show evidence of cardiac or respiratory failure should be referred for polysomnography to diagnose OSAS.
- Tonsillectomy/adenoidectomy is the first-line treatment for OSAS with continuous positive airway pressure an option for those unable to have surgery or for those who do not respond to surgical treatment.
- High-risk children should be monitored as inpatients after surgery.
- Re-evaluation is needed after surgery to determine effectiveness.

ATS Standards/Indications for Cardiopulmonary Sleep Studies in Children

The American Thoracic Society issued standards and indications for pediatric cardiopulmonary sleep studies to assist with the diagnosis of sleep-related breathing disorders (e.g., obstructive sleep apnea syndrome, OSAS) in children. Indications for polysomnography include:

- Differentiating benign snoring or primary snoring from pathological snoring that involves periods of apnea.
- Evaluating children who experience disturbances in patterns of sleep, including waking sleepiness, who fail to thrive, or who exhibit cor pulmonale or polycythemia, especially in children who snore.
- Clarifying clinical observations and diagnosis.
- Evaluating children with laryngomalacia and stridor (worsening at night).
- Evaluating the effects of obesity if other symptoms, such as snoring, sleep disturbance, or hypercapnia, are present.
- Evaluating the condition of the child with sickle cell disease with evidence of OSAS or veno-occlusive disease.
- Noting progress after treatment (4 weeks postsurgical) or weight loss (if indicated to control OSAS).
- Administering the multiple sleep latency test to evaluate excessive daytime sleepiness if OSAS is not noted.
- Assisting with titrating continuous positive airway pressure in those with OSAS.

The American Thoracic Society has established recommendations regarding polysomnography for a number of childhood disorders.

Bronchopulmonary dysplasia	Children may receive supplemental oxygen to maintain oxygen saturation at more than 92%.

35

	Assess oxygen saturation levels during both waking and sleeping hours to determine if hypoxemia occurs. Assess oxygen saturation levels after oxygen is discontinued if unexplained symptoms occur, such as cor pulmonale, polycythemia, and failure to thrive. Evaluate bradycardia occurring without apnea and snoring or suspected upper airway obstruction. Evaluate gastric reflux disease (pH sensor).
Cystic fibrosis	Provide continuous nocturnal oximetry if daytime oxygen saturation level is less than 95%.
	Use nocturnal oximetry for at least 8 hours if child has headaches in the morning, cor pulmonale, polycythemia, or daytime sleepiness. Diagnose OSAS in a child receiving supplemental oxygen with symptoms of cor pulmonale, polycythemia, and decrease in nocturnal oxygen saturation.
	Determine adverse effects of supplemental oxygen in the presence of severe lung disease.
Asthma	Do a polysomnography with pH sensor if nocturnal symptoms may be related to gastroesophageal reflux disease.
	Use nocturnal oximetry for children who experience asthma attacks during the night, complain of headaches on awakening, or have other types of disturbed sleep or cor pulmonale.
Neuro-muscular disorders (e.g., muscular dystrophy, cerebral palsy)	Do a polysomnography with end-tidal or transcutaneous carbon dioxide monitoring: If respiratory muscles are weak and forced vital capacity is less than 40%, PIP is less than 15 cm H_2O, or child has difficulty swallowing. If impairment is beyond that expected by diagnosis occurs, including snoring, cor pulmonale, headache on awakening, failure to thrive, and delay in development. As part of planning for nocturnal mechanical ventilation. For evaluation of respiratory treatment and care. As preoperative or postoperative assessment.
Alveolar hypoventilation syndrome	Polysomnography with carbon dioxide monitoring is indicated: To determine severity of disorder. To evaluate condition/treatment (periodically). To evaluate clinically unstable children with symptoms that include cor pulmonale, polycythemia, failure to thrive, developmental delay, headaches upon awakening, or altered mental status.
Infantile apnea/ bradycardia	While polysomnography is not recommended for routine evaluation of infants with apnea/bradycardia experiencing an apparent life-threatening event, it may be indicated: To clarify the frequency of apnea and type and alterations in the EEG, ECG and other parameters, especially if OSAS or ineffective control of respiration is suspected or bradycardia occurs without central apnea.

Abbreviations: EEG = electroencephalogram, ECG = electrocardiogram; and OSAS = obstructive sleep apnea syndrome.

MONITORING OF AHI AND INDICATIONS FOR UARS

Apnea-hypopnea index (AHI)	AHI is the total of apneic and hypopneic events in 1 hour of sleep. Apnea is absence of breathing while hypopnea is ineffectual or inadequate breathing, with exchange of air about 25%-70% of normal. The AHI for obstructive sleep apnea (OSA) is 15 or more.
Upper airway resistance syndrome (UARS)	UARS is characterized by an AHI of 5 or less but with increased numbers of respiratory effort-related arousals (RERAs) because of airway resistance to breathing during sleep caused by small, restricted airways. While snoring is a common indicator of upper airway collapse and OSA, the elimination of apneic periods and snoring alone does not indicate adequate titration for UARS. Rather, the focus must be on elimination of RERAs as well because some patients, especially women, have UARS without snoring. The oronasal thermistors normally used to evaluate airflow may not be sufficient to diagnose RERAs in UARS because RERAs may be less obvious; instead, esophageal cannulas with pressure transducers may be needed to show a reduction in flow.

MONITORING OF RERAS AND RDI

Respiratory effort-related arousals (RERAs)	RERAs typically occur when the patient falls asleep and begins snoring as muscle tone decreases, allowing the upper airway to collapse. The central nervous system senses apnea and responds by increasing muscle tone, blood pressure, and the metabolic rate. These changes cause the person to arouse enough to trigger inspiration, at which point the patient usually falls back to sleep. RERAs may occur many times during the night, preventing the person from falling into a deep sleep and resulting in chronic sleepiness.
Respiratory disturbance index (RDI)	RDI is the total of all respiratory disturbance events, including apnea and hypopnea as well as snoring, arousals, desaturation, and hypoventilation in 1 hour. In some cases, the apnea-hypopnea index and the RDI may be identical, but in other cases the RDI will be higher. The RDI is used to determine the severity of sleeping disorders: Normal =< 5 Mild = 5 − 20 Moderate = 20 − 40 Severe => 40

EXCESSIVE DAYTIME SLEEPINESS AND FATIGUE

Excessive daytime sleepiness (EDS), an increasing societal problem related to lack of adequate sleep, causes the patient to feel sleepy during waking hours to the point at which the person may fall asleep or feel the need to nap.

Fatigue, on the other hand, is a general feeling of tiredness, weakness, or lack of energy and may be related to physical or emotional problems. A person who is fatigued generally does not feel sleepy

or have difficulty staying awake. Patients often do not distinguish between sleepiness and fatigue, so the technician should question patients carefully to determine which they are experiencing:

- **EDS:** "Do you feel the need to sleep during the daytime?" "Do you feel drowsy?"
- **Fatigue:** "Do you feel as though you have no energy?" "Do you feel weary or weak?"

Sleepiness and fatigue scales may also be administered to help with diagnosis. Patients should evaluate sleepiness and fatigue at different times of the day with 9 am and 9 pm usually the time when people are most alert and 3 pm the least.

MSLT

The multiple sleep latency test (MSLT) measures sleepiness during waking hours and the tendency of a person to fall asleep. The MSLT may diagnose narcolepsy and idiopathic hypersomnia and determine the effectiveness of therapy. Elements include:

- Patient keeps a 2-week sleep diary before testing, sometimes with actigraphy, to identify sleeping patterns.
- Medications are assessed and withheld when possible if they affect sleep. Stimulants should be discontinued for 2 weeks before testing.
- The MSLT must be preceded by nocturnal polysomnography, and the montage includes electroencephalogram, electrooculogram, chin electromyogram, and electrocardiogram.
- MSLT includes five nap periods with first within 3 hours of a nocturnal polysomnogram and then spaced at 2 hours after start of preceding nap.
- Patients report their subjective evaluation of sleepiness 45 minutes before five designated nap periods, and physiological calibrations are done 5 minutes before onset of nap period.
- No smoking is allowed within 30 minutes of starting a nap and no strenuous activity within 15 minutes.
- Mean sleep latency is evaluated.

MWT

The maintenance of wakefulness test (MWT), done to assess sleepiness and effectiveness of treatment, determines the patient's ability to stay awake in the daytime. The MWT may be done with the multiple sleep latency test (MSLT). Elements include:

- A 2-week sleep diary and nocturnal polysomnogram may be done before the MWT, depending on the patient.
- Montage is similar to the MSLT: electroencephalogram, electrooculogram, chin electromyogram, and electrocardiogram.
- Patient is placed at rest, sitting in bed with low lights for four 40-minute periods, spaced at 2 hours, and advised to remain awake but not to engage in activities (e.g., singing, moving).
- Sleep latency (onset of sleep) is measured with fewer than 8 minutes considered abnormal. About half of normal sleepers remain awake during all 40-minute periods.
- Patient is awakened 90 seconds after falling asleep as duration of sleep is not important for the MWT alone.
- If the patient does not fall asleep during the 40-minute resting period, the test is terminated.

SUBJECTIVE SLEEPINESS EVALUATIONS

Subjective sleepiness evaluations, using various scales, are sometimes provided by the patient. While these evaluations are easy to use, take little time, and are usually available at no cost in print or online, the results should not be considered definitive because of a number of inherent weaknesses:

- Patients do not always report truthfully.
- Different scales measure different things and may not correlate.
- Some patients may receive a false positive and some a false negative.
- Scales are by their nature not objective so they are open to interpretation.
- The scales do not reflect comorbid conditions.
- People from different ethnic backgrounds may perceive sleep, sleepiness, and fatigue in different ways.
- Men and women may perceive sleep, sleepiness, and fatigue in different ways.

STANFORD SLEEPINESS SCALE

The Stanford Sleepiness Scale is a brief assessment used to determine if people have excessive daytime sleepiness (EDS). The scale is used at a number of different times during the day as people may report feeling sleepy at different times, especially in the late afternoon, a low period of alertness for most people. The scale lists seven descriptors that rate increasing levels of sleepiness. People with an EDS score of 4-7 have a sleep debt that interferes with functioning:

1 = Fully alert and awake
2 = Functioning and concentrating well but slightly sluggish.
3 = Awake and functioning but not fully alert
4 = Slightly foggy
5 = Foggy, slightly drowsy
6 = Feeling sleepy and drowsy and having difficulty staying awake
7 = Nearing onset of sleep and awake dreaming
X = Sleeping

EPWORTH SLEEPINESS SCALE

The Epworth Sleepiness Scale evaluates how likely a person is to fall asleep during a number of different activities. The person rates each situation on a scale of 0-3, corresponding to the chance of falling asleep (none, slight, moderate, or high). Situations queried include the following:

- Sitting and reading.
- Watching television.
- Sitting quietly in a public place, such as a meeting, movie, or theater.
- Sitting as a passenger in a car for an hour or more with no break.
- Lying down for an afternoon rest.
- Sitting and visiting with someone.
- Sitting quietly after eating lunch (which did not include alcohol).
- Sitting in a car while stopped in traffic for a few minutes.

Scores are totaled with 1-6 indicating the person is receiving adequate sleep. The average score for most people is 7-8, but scores of 9 or higher indicate the person has a high index for sleepiness and should have further testing.

EXCESSIVE DAYTIME SLEEPINESS SUB-SCALE OF SWAI

The Sleep-Wake Activity Inventory (SWAI) is a comprehensive instrument that includes subscales that measure a number of different aspects of sleep disorders: excessive daytime sleepiness (EDS), nocturnal sleep, relaxing ability, energy, social desirability, and psychological distress. The **EDS subscale** asks the patient to score nine different statements about sleepiness on 1-9 scale (always present to never present). Descriptors include:

- I fall asleep while watching television.
- I am able to nap anywhere.
- I fall asleep in the middle of a conversation.
- I feel drowsy within a few minutes while driving.
- I feel drowsy within 10 minutes of sitting quietly.
- I fall asleep during visits with friends.
- I feel sleepy after 15 minutes of reading.
- I fall asleep when I am relaxed.
- I fall asleep when I am riding in a car as a passenger.

Scores are added together. A score 50 or more is normal, but 40-50 suggests sleepiness, and a score of 40 or less indicates EDS.

FATIGUE SEVERITY SCALE

The Fatigue Severity Scale contains a list of nine descriptions related to fatigue. The patient scores each statement on a 1-7 scale (strongly disagree to strongly agree). Descriptors include:

- I have less motivation when I am fatigued.
- I become fatigued when I exercise.
- I become fatigued easily.
- My fatigue interferes with my ability to function physically.
- I experience frequent problems because of fatigue.
- I cannot carry out sustained physical activities/functioning because of fatigue.
- I cannot adequately carry out all of my duties and responsibilities because of fatigue.
- Fatigue is one of the three most disabling symptoms that I experience.
- My work, social, and family life suffer because of my fatigue.

The scores are added together with scores of 9-35 in the normal range and scores above 35 suggesting a high degree of fatigue.

HOME SLEEP APNEA TESTING

In-home sleep apnea testing can be performed on those patients who are suspected to have moderate to severe obstructive sleep apnea that do not have any chronic respiratory or cardiac medical conditions. Key elements of home sleep apnea testing include:

- Before doing an in-home test for sleep apnea, the patient will need to pick up the equipment or have it delivered to them, depending upon the office interpreting the test. They can be taught in person how to attach the sensors or printed instructions can be provided.
- It is important that the patient follow their regular routine so their sleep pattern will follow its normal cycle. Caffeine products should be avoided after mid-day and the patient should not take a nap during the day.
- At the patient's normal bedtime, they will attach the sensors to their body as instructed. Depending upon the equipment used, the patient will need to start the equipment to record the information over night. The sensors can be removed in the morning.
- The data collected by the machine is interpreted and forwarded to the ordering physician.

PROS AND CONS

Pros of home sleep apnea testing include:

- It is usually **less expensive** than sleep testing performed at a sleep center.
- It is **more convenient**, allowing the patient to sleep at home in their normal environment rather than in a different place.
- The equipment typically **requires fewer electrodes** and connections, so the patient can be more comfortable.
- There is **more access** to the testing because the patient does not need to travel to a sleep center, which may be far from their home.

Cons of home sleep apnea testing include:

- Home testing **does not include measurements** of sleep stages, heart rhythm with an EKG, and leg or arm movement sensors.
- Home tests may not be able to diagnose mild sleep apnea.
- Because the patient is applying the equipment and sensors themselves, there is the possibility that it may not be connected correctly, which can lead to **inadequate information.**
- If the information collected from a home test is inconclusive or not adequate, the sleep **study may need to be repeated at a sleep center** to ensure trained personnel are conducting the test.

Identify, Respond, and Document

WAVEFORM VARIATIONS

ALPHA WAVES

Alpha waves are 8-13 Hz frequency with an amplitude of less than 50 microvolts for adults, but often slightly slower for children and older adults. Alpha waves are slow and synchronous and are most typical at the onset of sleep when the patient is very drowsy and the eyes are closed. They also occur with deep relaxation and meditation. Alpha waves are suppressed when the eyes open. Alpha waves may also occur during arousals. Alpha waves are more noticeable in the occipital leads as they originate in the occipital cortex. Alpha-delta waves are slow alpha waves, occurring during periods of stage N3 sleep usually characterized by delta waves.

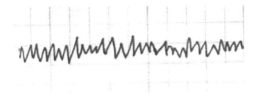

BETA WAVES

Beta waves are 13-35 Hz with an amplitude of less than 30 microvolts. Beta waves are present during normal wakefulness when the patient is alert.

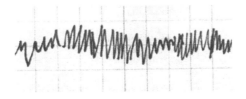

DELTA WAVES

Delta waves are slow 1-4 Hz with a high amplitude of more than 75 microvolts and are present in stage N3 (slow-wave) sleep in adults. Delta waves occur in the waking state of newborns and young children and may occur in adults who are intoxicated or have dementia or schizophrenia. Delta waves are involved in the release of human growth hormone, and patients are most deeply asleep during delta-wave activity.

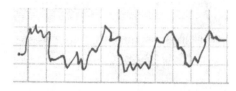

THETA WAVES

Theta waves are 4-6 Hz with oscillations of varying amplitude and are most easily observed with central and temporal leads. Theta waves are common during daydreaming and self-hypnotic states, occur in stage N1 sleep, and may occur during arousals.

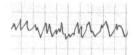

SAWTOOTH WAVES

Sawtooth waves are notched waves in the theta range that occur during stage R sleep and are most easily observed with frontal and vertex leads.

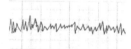

VERTEX WAVES

Vertex waves (vertex sharp transients, vertex sharp deflections, V waves) are commonly found negative deflections with amplitude usually ranging from 50-150 microvolts; they are most noticeable from vertex and frontal leads. They may have sharp contours and occur in repetitive episodes (especially in children).

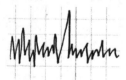

SLEEP SPINDLES

Sleep spindles are 12-14 Hz with an amplitude of less than 30 microvolts and a duration of 0.5-1.5 seconds, representing sudden bursts of electrical activity, usually most noticeable from central leads. They are slightly slower than alpha waves. Sleep spindles occur in sleep stages N2 and N3 but do not occur in stage N1 or R. Sleep spindles usually indicate the onset of stage N2. Similar appearing spindles may occur with benzodiazepine use, but they can be differentiated by a higher frequency (15 Hz).

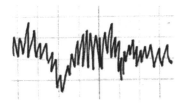

K COMPLEXES

K complexes are sharp negative waves (usually > 100 microvolts), preceding slower positive waves, and finally smaller negative waves, persisting for more than 0.5 seconds, sometimes followed by sleep spindles. K complexes occur during stage N2 sleep, usually every 1-1.7 minutes.

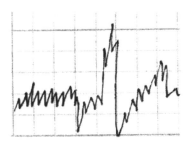

WICKET SPIKE WAVES

Wicket spike waves are 6-11 Hz frequency and occur primarily in older adults in a drowsy wake stage or stage N1 sleep. They are a normal variant and do not indicate pathology. Wicket spikes have a symmetric up and down arc and do not cross below the baseline as interictal epileptiform activity does, and they have little impact on the background electroencephalogram (EEG) reading. They may occur as single spikes or runs of spikes and are not followed by a slow wave.

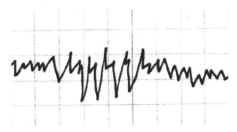

BENIGN EPILEPTIFORM TRANSIENTS OF SLEEP OR SMALL SHARP SPIKES

Benign epileptiform transients of sleep occur occasionally in stage N1 and N2 sleep. They are also called **small sharp spikes** because they are brief (< 50 milliseconds) with small amplitude (< 50 milliampere) and do not disrupt the background EEG.

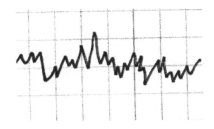

INTERICTAL EPILEPTIFORM ACTIVITY

Interictal epileptiform activity (IEA) is electrical discharges that occur between epileptic seizures. IEA usually occurs in brief bursts of electrical activity rather than the prolonged activity that is more representative of actual seizures. Typically, the spikes are asymmetric, with the downward arc, crossing below the baseline and more sloping than the upward arc. There are **four types,** which are described below.

Sharp wave	Pointed waves that are distinct from the background electroencephalogram, lasting 70-200 milliseconds
Spike	Similar to sharp-wave discharges but duration is shorter, 20-70 milliseconds.
Spike and slow-wave complex	Spike discharge followed by a slow wave of higher amplitude
Multiple spike and slow-wave complex	Multiple spike and slow-wave complex: multiple spikes (> 2) followed by one or more slow waves

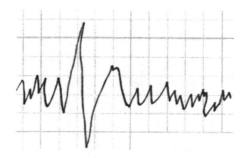

EPILEPTIC SEIZURE ACTIVITY

Epileptic seizure activity is evident on the polysomnogram (PSG), often across all channels, but the presentation depends on the type of seizure. Some seizure activity, such as frontal lobe epilepsy, occurs primarily during sleep. Seizure activity is most common during NREM sleep stages, especially stage N2. A PSG may help to differentiate between obstructive sleep apnea syndrome (OSAS) and frontal lobe epilepsy, which can result in similar symptoms of choking and excessive daytime drowsiness. In some cases, both epilepsy and OSAS may be present. Sleep disorders may exacerbate epileptic activity. Four-channel electroencephalogram recordings are more likely to demonstrate frontal lobe epilepsy accurately than temporal lobe, which is better identified with 18 channels, so some epileptic activity may be difficult to identify. Video monitoring during PSG can help to identify seizure activity, which usually involves some degree of arousal.

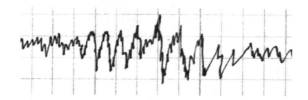

ARTIFACTS
IDENTIFICATION AND MONITORING

Artifacts, extraneous signals, are common during polysomnography; some relate to normal activity, such as muscle movement or snoring. The technician must monitor, identify, and correct artifacts as necessary by:

- Checking other channels to determine if the artifacts are occurring in only one channel or adjacent channels as well. If in only one channel, then the artifact may be related to a single lead.
- Determining if the affected channels share a reference lead as this suggests the artifact relates to the reference.
- Changing the derivation of the input signal, typically to the opposite side, so if C_4 shows artifacts, change to C_3.
- Monitoring constantly and change derivations as needed through system referencing or the use of multiple channels.

LOW-LEVEL 50-60 HZ ARTIFACTS

Low-level 50-60 Hz artifacts from power line interference, other electrical equipment, or an electrode connection are commonly found in polysomnography and are often detected in electromyogram (EMG) channels, such as the chin EMG (cEMG). Additionally, especially if related to dislodged electrodes, the electrocardiogram (ECG) signals may be evident in the cEMG channel. In the case of 60 Hz artifacts, the appearance of the cEMG recording will be very uniform.

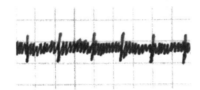

ELECTRODE POPPING/CHIN ELECTROMYOGRAM ARTIFACTS

Electrode popping causes a series of spike-like waves that mirror respirations, usually because the electrode is loose, dirty, faulty, or pressing against bedding. ECG signals may also be evident in the cEMG recording. A tight electrode seal to the skin may prevent electrode popping.

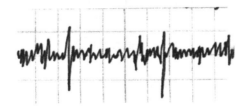

ARTIFACTS CAUSED BY AIRFLOW AND RESPIRATORY EFFORT SENSORS

Airflow and respiratory effort sensors can easily cause artifacts during polysomnography. An indication that airflow artifacts are present is when the nasal airflow is out of sync with the chest and abdominal airflow effort sensors. Respiratory effort recordings that are out of phase often indicate that one or more belts are too loose or too tight or have been dislodged by body movement. The sleep technologist must distinguish between recordings that indicate partial obstruction, which can result in out-of-phase respiratory effort recordings, and artifacts. Temperature-based and pressure-based sensors have different properties, so the technologist should be familiar with the properties and limitations of the sensors used when determining whether a recording represents an artifact.

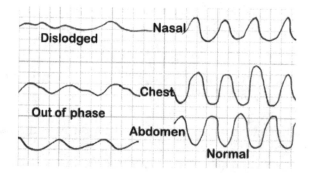

MOVEMENT ARTIFACTS

Movement artifacts can cause distortion of all channels and may involve a number of other overlapping artifacts, such as electrode popping and muscle artifacts. Movement artifacts may be difficult to control and may interfere with recordings for patients who are extremely restless or move frequently during sleep. Often, excessive movement artifacts relate to improper application of electrodes or pulling on electrode wires as the patient turns. Securing the electrodes and making sure that the wires can accommodate turning and moving can reduce movement artifacts.

MUSCLE ARTIFACTS

Muscle artifacts usually result from localized muscle activity near a reference or exploring electrode. Muscle artifacts can cause irregular distortion in multiple channels, such as the electroencephalogram and electrooculogram. Muscle artifacts can occur if a patient is extremely tense, so sometimes asking the patient to relax and slightly open the jaw can reduce artifacts. Artifacts may also relate to chewing movements or teeth grinding. In many cases, the electrodes should be re-referenced. The recording in the chin electromyogram is not considered an artifact because it is intended to measure muscle activity and normally increases with muscle tension or activity.

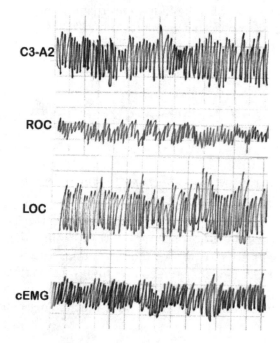

ELECTROCARDIOGRAM ARTIFACTS

Electrocardiogram (ECG) artifacts, recognizable by spikes that match the ECG recording in the electroencephalogram and electrooculogram channels, are common and not always avoidable, but they should not be prominent to the point that they obscure or confuse data. ECG artifacts are often more pronounced in obese patients, so reference electrodes should not be placed over soft fatty tissue. Double referencing the A1 and A2 reference electrodes can also minimize ECG artifacts; however, double referencing may cause increased interference from other types of artifacts, so double referencing should not be a routine procedure. ECG artifacts in the electromyogram channels usually indicate poor placement of electrodes or unequal impedances.

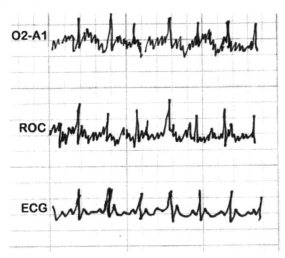

SLOW-FREQUENCY ARTIFACTS

Slow-frequency artifacts can be related to perspiration, pressure on an electrode, or body movement. Perspiration, the most common reason, results in chemical changes that cause a slow, frequently oscillating pattern that mirrors breathing patterns, often caused by small head movements with respirations. If caused by perspiration, lowering the temperature in the room by use of air conditioning or fans may help to resolve the problem. If caused by position, raising the low-frequency filter, changing the input derivation to the opposite side, or repositioning the patient may help. Careful and secure application of electrodes may decrease the incidence of slow-frequency artifacts.

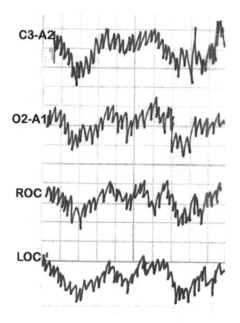

OXIMETRY ARTIFACTS

Oximetry artifacts must be monitored carefully because interference may result in inaccurate readings that impact the study results. Inaccurate recordings may result from improper application of the oximeter, displacement (often related to movement), poor perfusion in distal extremities, motion artifacts, or inaccurate calibrations. Obesity may also interfere with oximetry recordings. The technician should monitor the oximetry channel carefully and note irregular recordings, sudden variations, or abnormally low readings that do not correlate with other data. Oximetry artifacts must be tagged or removed from the recordings. Artifacts may be identified by noting changes in oxygen saturation in a consecutive series of sampling times. Pulse oximetry must always be correlated with other findings because pulse oximetry cannot identify sleep disorders that are unrelated to oxygen desaturation.

MECHANICAL ARTIFACTS

Mechanical artifacts can result from problems with equipment, including incorrect application or dislodging of electrodes and sensors.

Cause	Result	Correction
Condensation in CPAP tubing.	Fluid in tubing can cause M-shaped waveform in airflow channel.	Remove fluid from tubing.
Loose belt (sensors)	Tracings are flat despite evidence of movement or respirations.	Reapply belt correctly.
Misplacement of airflow sensor	Sensor does not record changes in temperature/airflow.	Reposition.
Electrodes, loose or improperly secured	High-frequency noise combined with high amplitude can slow activity.	Remove, reprep skin, and reattach electrode.

48

Cause	Result	Correction
Oximetry channel	Inaccurate recordings of oxygen saturation can result from improperly attached oximeter.	Check placement and ensure fingernail is free of polish.
ECG in EEG, EOG, or EMG channels	ECG tracing appears in other channels.	Re-reference (double reference) channels for EEG/EOG to reference leads A_1 and A_2. Ensure electrodes are correctly placed and attached. Avoid applying reference electrodes to fat, soft tissue. Use common mode rejection for EMG artifacts, or reattach EMG electrodes.
Electrode pop (sharp, spiking deflection)	Electrode pops are generally related to only one electrode but may be observed in multiple channels.	Remove, reprep skin, and reattach electrode. Pops may result from pressure on electrodes, dirty electrodes, or loose wires.
Cardio-ballistic (sensors)	Sensors (respiratory effort, airflow) pick up pulse waves from ECG.	Note and record; correction not usually possible.

Abbreviation: CPAP = continuous positive airway pressure.

RECORDING-RELATED ARTIFACTS

Recording-related artifacts may relate to choice of channels or filters as well as interference from equipment.

Cause	Result	Correction
50-60 Hz	Caused by poor grounding of EEG electrodes or interference from electrical leakage from other equipment; 50-60 Hz artifacts can occur in EMG channels, especially leg EMGs.	Use common mode rejection. A 50-60 notch filter may remove artifacts at 50-60 Hz, but do not use in EEG or EOG channels as artifacts there usually indicate improper connection.
Multiple channel recordings	Multiple source artifacts can make a recording unreadable, and multiple channels cannot be shown at the same time so important data may be missed.	Reconsider approach.
Excessive filtering	Filtering can distort data and mask problems that require correction.	Avoid using filters to reduce artifacts, and do not use filters to remove artifacts unless underlying physiological signals are adequate.

PHYSIOLOGICAL ARTIFACTS

Physiological artifacts can be caused by numerous factors (extraneous signals) that alter the results of polysomnography.

Cause	Result	Correction
Muscle (electromyogram EMG)	The background electroencephalogram (EEG) or electro-oculogram may be obscured and other signals distorted, depending on the type of muscle activity.	Encourage patient to relax, deep breathe, and slightly open the jaw to reduce tension. Report on visual observations when artifacts occur, noting signs of seizures or a sleep behavior disorder. Ensure electrodes are correctly attached.
Skin irritation (rash)	Irritation, such as a skin rash, can alter the skin's electrical signal, causing high impedance.	Place electrode in a different area, avoiding irritated skin.
Vibration	Leg movement or snoring can cause high-frequency artifacts.	Note and record all artifacts; correction is not usually possible.
Perspiration (EEG)	Excess perspiration may cause low-frequency artifacts.	Cool patient by changing room temperature or using fans.
Swallow (EEG)	Swallowing can result in slow waves in temporal areas, typical on arousal.	Note and record; correction not usually possible.
Retinal disease (EOG)	The affected eye may interfere with electrical signal.	Note activity of unaffected eye, or use other measures.
Artificial eye (EOG)	The prosthetic eye does not generate electrical signals.	Note underlying frontal EEG activity.
Blink (EOG)	Produces slow waves, depending on type and speed of activity.	Note and record; correction not usually possible.
Eye muscle abnormality (weakness, hyperactivity, paralysis) [EOG, EEG]	Abnormalities may alter EOG readings, depending on the type of abnormality. Rectus movement can cause spike in EEG (frontotemporal).	Note activity of unaffected eye or use other measures.

Abbreviations: EEG = electroencephalogram; and EOG = electrooculogram.

Physiologic/Clinical Events

RETICULAR FORMATION

The reticular formation, located in the brainstem, receives neural impulses from everywhere in the body and is connected to both the cerebellum, which controls movement, balance, and coordination, and the limbic system (deep brain structures).

- The **ascending pathways (dorsal and ventral),** referred to as the reticular activating system (RAS), carry sensory information to the forebrain and cerebral cortex, and use a feedback method to control sleep and awake states. Sensory input and activity in the RAS bring about arousal and maintain the awake state. The RAS is linked to the motor system and controls movement during the awake state and atonia during stage R sleep.
- The **descending reticular formation** receives input from the hypothalamus and is involved in activation of the autonomic nervous system.

NEUROTRANSMITTERS INVOLVED IN SLEEP

Neurotransmitters involved in sleep include the following:

Acetylcholine	Levels increase during the wake state and during stage R sleep, but levels decrease during stages N1, N2, and N3 sleep.
Adenosine	Levels increase during periods of sleep deprivation and decrease when sleeping to recover. Some drugs, such as theophylline and caffeine, suppress the function of adenosine.
Dopamine	Levels increase during the wake state and during stage R sleep. Some stimulants, such as methamphetamine, increase levels.
Gamma-aminobutyric acid	Levels increase to inhibit the central nervous system.
Glutamate	Levels increase to stimulate the central nervous system.
Glycine	Levels increase to inhibit the motor nervous system at the spinal cord to cause atonia during Stage R sleep.
Histamine	Levels increase during the wake state. Agents that block histamine-1 receptors increase drowsiness.
Hypocretin 1, 2	Levels increase during the wake state and regulate the circadian cycle. Impairment of hypocretin production or utilization can cause narcolepsy.
Immunomodulators with sleep factors	Levels increase non-REM sleep (insulin, interleukin I, interferon-α_2, tumor necrosis factor).
	Levels increase REM sleep (somatostatin, growth hormone, prolactin).
	Levels increase both non-REM and REM sleep (prostaglandin D2, growth hormone-releasing factor).
	Levels inhibit sleep (glucocorticoids, prostaglandin E2, corticotropin-releasing factor, thyrotropin-releasing hormone).
Melatonin	Levels increase during the evening and night and begin to decrease in the morning, helping to control the sleep-wake cycle.
Norepinephrine	Levels increase to maintain the awake state, so levels decrease during stages N1, N2, and N3 sleep and are absent in stage R sleep.
Serotonin	Levels increase during the awake state but decrease during non-REM and REM sleep to help regulate sleep onset with lowest levels during REM.

PATHOPHYSIOLOGY OF SLEEP

LIMBIC SYSTEM

The limbic system, in the region of the diencephalon, is essential to regulation of emotion, hormones, mood, and pain or pleasure sensations. The limbic system is comprised of several structures, including:

- **Amygdala:** This is an almond-shaped grouping of nuclei that are responsible for mediating arousal, emotion, and fear responses, as well as hormones.
- **Cingulate gyrus:** This structure is responsible for matching sensory input with emotional response.
- **Hippocampus:** This is a group of neurons responsible for organizing and processing memories, spatial relationships, and emotional regulation.
- **Hypothalamus:** This is a structure that is involved in almost all body processes, to include autonomic functions, emotions, homeostasis, endocrine processes, and sleep regulation.
- **Thalamus:** This is a group of cells that mediates motor function, and receives, processes, and relays sensory signals to and from the cortex, playing an important role in sleep. Fibers release neurotransmitters that help to control arousal.

DIENCEPHALON

The diencephalon is located above the brainstem and between the cerebral hemispheres. It comprises primarily gray matter and surrounds the third ventricle. The diencephalon contains a number of structures important to sleep and arousal.

- **Thalamus:** This gland receives sensory input from other parts of the central nervous system and carries them to appropriate areas of the cerebral cortex. The thalamus serves as a gateway and also an editor for sensory input (except for smell).
- **Hypothalamus:** This gland regulates heart rate, blood pressure, temperature, fluid and electrolyte balance, hunger, weight, stomach, intestines, and sleep; and produces substances that stimulate the pituitary gland to release hormones.
- **Optic chiasm:** The optic nerves cross in this area anterior to the pituitary gland.
- **Posterior pituitary gland:** This gland stores and secretes oxytocin and antidiuretic hormone, which are produced by the hypothalamus.
- **Mamillary bodies:** These are active in the memory of smells.
- **Pineal gland:** This gland is attached to the third ventricle; it produces melatonin and mediates sleep.

RESPIRATORY SYSTEM DURING AWAKE STAGE

The respiratory system during the awake stage is under primary control of the autonomic nervous system. However, speaking and eating can interfere with respirations, and they can also be controlled voluntarily, such as when a person holds his or her breath. The upper respiratory tract, including the nose, nasal passages, sinuses, pharynx, tonsils, adenoids, larynx, and trachea, warms, filters, and moistens the air that is inhaled, but obstruction of the upper respiratory tract may interfere with this function and cause people to become mouth breathers. While breathing through the mouth occurs with exercise, chronic mouth breathing can cause dryness of the mucous membranes in the mouth and can result in abnormalities of facial growth in children. The lower respiratory tract (the lungs) accomplishes gas exchange, that is, oxygen for carbon dioxide.

RESPIRATORY TERMINOLOGY FOR LUNG VOLUMES AND CAPACITY

Respiratory terminology for lung volumes and lung capacities includes the following:

Tidal volume	Amount of air exchange with each breath (500 mL/kg for adults or 5-10 mL/kg for infants and children).
Residual volume	Amount of air remaining in the lungs after a forced exhalation. Average for adults is 1200 mL, but this may increase with chronic obstructive pulmonary disease (COPD).
Vital capacity	The maximal amount of air exhaled after maximal inhalation. Average for adults is 4600 mL; it decreases with neuromuscular disease, atelectasis, and fatigue.
Functional residual capacity	The amount of air remaining in the lungs after a normal exhalation; the average for adults is 2300 mL, but this may increase with COPD and decrease with acute respiratory distress syndrome.
Total lung capacity	The amount of air in the lungs after a maximal inhalation. Average for adults is 5800 mL, but this may increase with COPD and decrease with pneumonia or atelectasis.

PRIMARY RESPIRATORY FUNCTION

The primary respiratory function is to facilitate the body's cells to obtain energy from the oxidation of carbohydrates, fats, and proteins, a process that requires oxygen and generates carbon dioxide as a by-product.

Oxygen transport	Blood circulates to carry oxygen to the cells and to remove carbon dioxide by diffusion at the capillary level.
Respiration	Gas exchange occurs between the atmospheric air and the blood and between the blood and the body cell.
	The capillaries in the lungs have a lower concentration of oxygen than the alveoli, so oxygen diffuses into the blood.
	The capillaries have a higher concentration of carbon dioxide than the alveoli, so carbon dioxide diffuses into the alveoli.
Ventilation	Air flows into the lungs during inspiration and back into the atmosphere during expiration with airflow governed by variances in air pressure, airway resistance, and compliance.

VENTILATION

Ventilation carries air with oxygen into the lungs and waste products, including carbon dioxide, out of the lungs. Important factors include **air pressure variances** and **airway resistance**.

Air pressure variances:

- **Inspiration:** The thorax expands and lowers the pressure in the thoracic cavity relative to atmospheric pressure, drawing air into the alveoli.
- **Expiration:** The diaphragm relaxes, and the lungs contract; pressure inside the alveoli increases relative to atmospheric pressure, causing air to flow out of the lungs.

Airway resistance:

Resistance directly relates to the size of the airway, so changes in size can increase resistance, requiring an increased effort of breathing:

- Bronchial contraction of smooth muscles (asthma)
- Mucosal hyperplasia (chronic bronchitis)
- Airway obstruction (tumor, mucus, foreign body)
- Dilation or loss of elasticity as with chronic obstructive pulmonary disease (COPD)

COMPLIANCE

Ventilation carries air with oxygen into the lungs and waste products, including carbon dioxide, out of the lungs. An important factor is **compliance**. The elasticity and expandability of the lungs and thoracic cavity determine the volume/pressure relationship:

- Compliance decreases when lung expansion is limited or "tight" (pneumothorax, pulmonary edema, atelectasis), requiring increased effort of breathing.
- Compliance increases with overdistention of the thorax or loss of elasticity as in COPD.

HYPOXIC DRIVE

Respirations are primarily controlled by the level of arterial carbon dioxide ($PaCO_2$) rather than the level of oxygen (PaO_2). As carbon dioxide levels rise, this normally triggers an increased rate of respiration to compensate. In some cases, such as at high altitude, respirations can be triggered by hypoxemia; this is known as **hypoxic drive** because the concentration of ambient oxygen is lower. This same hypoxic drive can be triggered by patients with chronic hypercarbia (≤ 70 torr). Thus, when supplementary oxygen is delivered, the hypoxic drive, which has been triggering respirations, may decrease, resulting in hypopnea or apnea. Patients who are hypoxemic may still require oxygen, but administration must be carefully managed and the patient observed for changes in respiratory rate and effort. Patients with chronic obstructive pulmonary disease receiving high fractions of inspired oxygen may actually have increased carbon dioxide levels.

RESPIRATORY SYSTEM DURING STAGES N1, N2, N3, AND R

The respiratory system during stages N1, N2, N3 and R is completely under the control of the autonomic nervous system and is not impacted by activities of the awake state; thus, respirations should become very regular in both the respiratory rate and the amplitude:

- **Stages N1 and N2:** Some periodic breathing (irregular respirations with brief periods of apnea-hypopnea) may occur at sleep onset and throughout stage N1 but should disappear by stage N2. Periodic breathing is common with congestive heart failure.
- **Stage N3:** Respirations should remain regular with some decrease noted in tidal volume and functional residual capacity as well as a decrease in minute ventilation. $PaCO_2$ increases, and PaO_2 decreases. Inspiratory airflow decreases, and upper airway resistance increases. Muscle activity (muscles of respiration) decreases.

RESPIRATORY SYSTEM DURING STAGE R SLEEP

The respiratory system during stage R sleep changes as respirations become much more irregular in rate, amplitude, and tidal volume. Periodic breathing or central apneas (10-30 seconds) may occur during phasic REM sleep. Muscle hypotonia/atonia may affect the muscles of respiration, including the intercostals, and this can increase hypoventilation in patients with pulmonary disorders. The diaphragm muscle remains innervated by phrenic motor neurons, so it can

54

compensate for the loss of other muscle function; however, if the diaphragm is impaired, such as with neuromuscular disease, then hypoventilation occurs. The $PaCO_2$ increases by 2-5 mm Hg while the PaO_2 and functional residual capacity decrease, increasing hypoxemia in patients with sleep-disordered breathing because the compensatory ventilatory response is depressed. Upper airway resistance increases during stage R sleep and can lead to collapse of the airway and obstructive sleep apnea syndrome.

SNORING

Snoring results from vibration within the respiratory system, often within the throat or nasal passages. The sound arises from the tissues vibrating against each other. Causes can include the following:

- Throat muscle weakness.
- Obesity.
- Nasal obstruction.
- Tissues touching.
- Drug use (alcohol or other muscle relaxant drugs).
- Supine position (the tongue may obstruct the airway).

Snoring increases during sleep because the muscles relax, causing partial closure of the airway. Usually, the more the restriction in airflow, the louder the snoring. If related to nasal obstruction only (primary), snoring is usually regular and periodic and may be soft to loud. While annoying, this type of snoring is not a threat to health. Snoring related to obstructive sleep apnea is more irregular in rhythm and interrupted by periods of apnea-hypopnea and brief arousals. Patients may complain of headache on arising and chronic drowsiness.

CARDIOVASCULAR SYSTEM DURING SLEEP

The **cardiovascular system during sleep** responds to the control of both the sympathetic and parasympathetic nervous systems, causing changes in heart rate and blood pressure, although stroke volume usually remains constant with the lowest cardiac output during the final stage R sleep cycle. The changes can cause cardiovascular ischemia in some individuals:

- **Stages N1, N2, and N3 sleep:** For most patients, the parasympathetic nervous system is primary, causing a decrease in both the heart rate and blood pressure (decreased peripheral vascular resistance) by 5%-15%.
- **Stage R sleep:** During the phasic stage of REM sleep, the sympathetic nervous system affects the cardiovascular system by increasing both the heart rate and blood pressure (increased peripheral vascular resistance). However, during tonic REM sleep, the parasympathetic nervous system again lowers the heart rate, sometimes to bradycardic levels, and blood pressure.
- **Arousal response:** The sympathetic nervous system is involved in arousals, increasing heart rate and blood pressure.

CARDIAC OUTPUT

Cardiac output is the amount of blood pumped through the ventricles during a specified period. Oxygen must be delivered to the cells to prevent tissue and organ damage, so oxygen delivery should be continuously assessed by the technician. Normal cardiac output is about 5 L/min at rest for an adult. Under exercise or stress, this volume may multiply three or four times with concomitant changes in the heart rate (HR) and stroke volume (SV). The basic formulation for calculating cardiac output (CO) is the heart rate per minute multiplied by the stroke volume, which is the amount of blood pumped through the ventricles with each contraction. The stroke volume is controlled by preload (elasticity/volume of ventricles), afterload (systemic vascular resistance), and contractibility:

$$CO = HR/min \times SV.$$

The heart rate is controlled by the autonomic nervous system. Normally, if the heart rate decreases, stroke volume increases to compensate, but with cardiomyopathies, this may not occur, so bradycardia results in a sharp decline in cardiac output.

HEMODYNAMICS

Hemodynamics is based on the principle that fluid flows from areas of higher pressure to areas of lower pressure:

- **Systole:** Pressure rises in the ventricles, closing tricuspid and mitral (atrioventricular) valves, stopping flow from the atria and preventing backflow (regurgitation). Pressure forces the pulmonic and aortic valves (semilunar valves) open, sending blood into both the aorta and pulmonary artery. Early ventricular systolic pressure is high and then falls near the end of systole as the ventricles empty, lowering the pressure in the aorta and pulmonary artery, causing atrioventricular valves to close.
- **Diastole:** Ventricles are relaxed and atrioventricular valves open. Pressure in the atria is lower than in the venae cavae or pulmonary veins, pulling blood into the atria with some to the ventricles. An electrical impulse is generated in the sinoatrial node, forcing the atria to contract, increasing the pressure and forcing more blood through the valves and into the ventricles. This period is atrial systole and occurs near the end of ventricular diastole.

HEMODYNAMIC TERMS

Cardiac output (CO) is the amount of blood pumped through the ventricles, usually calculated in liters per minute. Normal value at rest are 4-6 L/min.

Cardiac index (CI) is the cardiac output divided by the body surface area (BSA) [CI = CO divided by BSA]. This is essentially a measure of cardiac output tailored to the individual, based on height and weight, measured in liters per minute per square meter of body surface area. Normal values are 2.2-4.0 L/min/m².

Stroke volume (SV) is the amount of blood pumped through the left ventricle with each contraction, minus any blood remaining inside the ventricle at the end of systole. Normal values are 60-70 mL. The formula is below:

(CO L/min) / ((HR/min) x (1000)) = SV mL

Pulmonary vascular resistance (PVR) is the resistance in the pulmonary arteries and arterioles against which the right ventricle has to pump during contraction. It is the mean pressure in the pulmonary vascular bed divided by blood flow. If PVR increases, SV decreases. Normal values are 1.2-3.0 units or 100-250 dynes/sec/cm⁵.

ARTERIAL OXYGEN

Arterial oxygen is carried in the red blood cells by hemoglobin. Each hemoglobin molecule can carry four molecules of oxygen, with 1 g of hemoglobin equal to 1.39 mL of oxygen (100 mL arterial blood carries 0.3 mL oxygen). When the hemoglobin is fully saturated (four oxygen molecules per molecule of hemoglobin), then arterial oxygen saturation is 100%. A small amount of oxygen remains dissolved in blood (PaO_2 x 0.0031), but this has little effect on arterial oxygen content. The **formula to determine arterial oxygen (CaO_2)** is below:

$$CaO_2 = [\text{hemoglobin x arterial oxygen saturation } (SaO_2) \text{ x } 1.39] + [\text{arterial partial pressure of oxygen} (PaO_2 \text{ x } 0.003].$$

Within the sleep laboratory, a simplified formula is used to evaluate oxygen delivery (O_2D):

$$O_2D = [\text{stroke volume x heart rate}] \text{ x } SpO_2.$$

Perfusion pressure is estimated by the systolic blood pressure:

$$\text{Systolic blood pressure} = \text{cardiac output x systemic vascular resistance.}$$

ARTERIAL BLOOD GASES

Arterial blood gases are sometimes monitored to assess the effectiveness of oxygenation, ventilation, and acid-base status and to determine oxygen flow rates. Partial pressure of a gas is that exerted by each gas in a mixture of gases, proportional to its concentration, based on total atmospheric pressure of 760 mm Hg at sea level. Normal arterial blood gas values include the following:

- Acidity/alkalinity (pH): 7.35-7.45
- Partial pressure of carbon dioxide ($PaCO_2$): 35-45 mm Hg
- Partial pressure of oxygen (PaO_2): ≥ 80 mg Hg
- Bicarbonate concentration (HCO_3): 22-26 mEq/L
- Oxygen saturation (SaO_2): ≥ 95%

The relationship between these elements, particularly the $PaCO_2$ and the PaO_2 indicates respiratory status. For example, $PaCO_2$ over 55 mm Hg and the PaO_2 under 60 mm Hg in a patient previously in good health indicates respiratory failure. There are many issues to consider. Ventilator management may require a higher $PaCO_2$ to prevent barotrauma and a lower PaO_2 to reduce oxygen toxicity.

> **Review Video: Blood Gases**
> Visit mometrix.com/academy and enter code: 611909

VENTILATION-PERFUSION

Ventilation-perfusion refers to oxygen diffusing across the alveolar membrane into the capillary blood. As oxygen in its gaseous form is exposed to the liquid blood, the oxygen dissolves until it reaches a state of equilibrium in which the partial pressure of the dissolved oxygen in the blood is equal to the partial pressure of oxygen in its gaseous state in the alveoli:

- **Normal ventilation-perfusion:** With normal lung function, blood passing by the alveoli is matched with an equal amount of gas, so ventilation matches perfusion (ratio 1:1).
- **Low ventilation-perfusion:** Shunting occurs when perfusion exceeds ventilation so that an adequate volume of blood passes by the alveoli, but the blood does not pick up adequate amounts of gas because of obstruction, such as from atelectasis.

- **High ventilation-perfusion:** Dead space occurs because ventilation is adequate but not blood supply so gas exchange is impaired. This can occur with pulmonary embolism and shock.
- **Silent unit:** No or very little exchange occurs, such as with pneumothorax or acute respiratory distress syndrome.

OXYHEMOGLOBIN DISSOCIATION CURVE

The **oxyhemoglobin dissociation curve** is a graph that plots the percentage of hemoglobin saturated with oxygen (y axis) and different partial pressures of oxygen (PaO_2 levels) [x axis]. A curve shift to the right represents conditions where hemoglobin has less affinity for oxygen (greater amounts of oxygen are released). A shift to the left has the opposite implications. Low pH shifts the curve to the right, enabling increased unloading of hemoglobin to tissues. Elevated oxygen shifts the curve to the left, causing increased affinity of hemoglobin for oxygen in the lungs. Small changes in fetal PO_2 result in greater loading or unloading of oxygen compared to adult hemoglobin. Because of the increased affinity for oxygen, lower tissue oxygen levels are needed to trigger the unload of oxygen. Thus, the infant will have a lower PaO_2 and oxygen saturation before cyanosis is evident. Normal PaO_2 is 80-100 mm Hg, equal to 95%-98% oxygen saturation. Levels less than 40 mm Hg are dangerous.

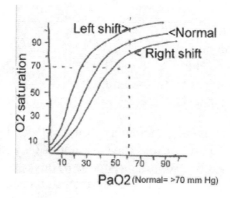

HEMOGLOBIN AND HEMATOCRIT

Hemoglobin and hematocrit are particularly important in evaluating the amount of oxygen in the blood. Red blood cells (RBCs or erythrocytes) contain hemoglobin (95% of mass), which carries oxygen throughout the body. The heme portion of the cell contains iron, which binds to the oxygen.

- **Hemoglobin**, a protein found in erythrocytes, uses iron to bind and transport oxygen. Deficiencies of amino acids, vitamins, or minerals can cause a decrease, impacting healing and reducing oxygen to tissue. Dehydration and severe burns can cause an increase. Normal values for men are 13-18 g/dL, and for women, 12-16 g/dL.
- **Hematocrit** measures the percentage of packed red blood cells in 100 mL of blood. A decrease can indicate blood loss and anemia. An increase may indicate dehydration, and measurements may monitor the effects of rehydration. Normal values for men are 42%-52%, and for women, 37%-48%.

GASTROINTESTINAL TRACT DURING SLEEP

The **gastrointestinal tract during sleep** slows down as a protective mechanism to prevent aspiration. Less saliva is produced, esophageal motility decreases, and the patient swallows less; however, the production of gastric acid increases during the night (peaking from 10 pm to 2 am) in response to stimulation of the parasympathetic nervous system. Stomach emptying slows during sleep. These changes pose a problem for patients with gastroesophageal reflux disease (GERD) because the increased acid flows back into the esophagus at the same time that clearance of secretions in the esophagus slows. This increases the risk of obstructive sleep apnea. Arousal, in turn, stimulates swallowing. Gastric peristalsis decreases during stages N1, N2, and N3 sleep but not in stage R sleep, resulting in fewer episodes of GERD during stage R sleep. Pain or discomfort related to gastrointestinal disorders can disrupt sleep significantly. It is likely that GERD will increase during sleep if the patient lies in the right lateral decubitus position.

IDENTIFYING AND RESPONDING TO EMERGENCIES

UNSTABLE AND VARIANT ANGINA

Unstable angina (also known as preinfarction or crescendo angina) is a progression of coronary artery disease and occurs when there is a change in the pattern of stable angina. The pain may increase, may not respond to a single nitroglycerin, and may persist for 5 minutes or more. Usually pain is more frequent, lasts longer, and may occur at rest. Unstable angina may indicate rupture of an atherosclerotic plaque and the beginning of thrombus formation so it should always be treated as a medical emergency as it may indicate a myocardial infarction.

Variant angina (also known as Prinzmetal's angina) results from spasms of the coronary arteries, either with or without atherosclerotic plaques, and is often related to smoking, alcohol, or illicit stimulants. Elevation of ST segments usually occurs with variant angina. Variant angina frequently occurs cyclically at the same time each day and often while the person is at rest, so it may occur during polysomnography.

MYOCARDIAL INFARCTION

Myocardial infarction (MI) occurs when there is an imbalance between the heart's demand for oxygen and the supply. An MI may occur after an episode of unstable angina caused by rupture of an atherosclerotic plaque and thrombosis associated with coronary artery spasm, but it may also result from vasoconstriction, acute blood loss, decreased oxygen, and cocaine ingestion. Symptoms of MI vary considerably, with men having the more "classic" symptom of sudden crushing chest pain and women and those under 55 presenting with atypical symptoms. Diabetic patients may have a reduced sensation of pain because of neuropathy, complaining primarily of weakness. Elderly patients may also have neuropathic changes that reduce the sensation of pain. Symptoms may include blood pressure changes, palpitations, angina, dyspnea, pulmonary or peripheral edema, pallor, cold clammy skin, and diaphoresis. Polysomnography may show changes in respiration, electrocardiographic changes (e.g., ST segment and T-wave changes, tachycardia, bradycardia, and dysrhythmias), and decreased oxygen saturation with hypoxia. Patient may need oxygen or cardiopulmonary resuscitation. Emergency assistance should be requested.

ACUTE ASTHMA ATTACK

An **acute asthma attack** is precipitated by some stimulus, such as an antigen that triggers an allergic response, resulting in an inflammatory cascade that causes edema of the mucous membranes (swollen airway), contraction of smooth muscles (bronchospasm), increased mucus production (cough and obstruction), and hyperinflation of airways (decreased ventilation and shunting). While asthma is more common in children, older adults are also affected but may be misdiagnosed. Older adults may complain of daytime sleepiness and increased asthma symptoms during the night, characterized by wheezing, dyspnea, and coughing. In cough-variant asthma, a severe cough may be the only symptom, at least initially. Bronchodilators should be available to relieve symptoms as patients may become hypoxic. With chronic asthma, permanent damage to airways may cause decreased oxygen saturation during sleep and disordered sleep. If nocturnal hypoxia is severe, the patient may require supplemental oxygen (1-2 L/min).

59

STROKE

Strokes (cerebrovascular accidents) result from interruption of the blood flow to an area of the brain. About 80% of strokes are ischemic, resulting from blockage of an artery supplying the brain because of thrombosis in a large artery, lacunar infarct (penetrating thrombosis in small artery), or embolism. Hemorrhagic strokes result from a ruptured cerebral artery, causing not only a lack of oxygen and nutrients but also edema that causes widespread pressure and damage. Strokes most commonly occur in the right or left hemisphere, but the exact location and the extent of brain damage affects the type of presenting symptoms. If the frontal area of either side is involved, there tends to be memory and learning deficits. Typical presenting symptoms include slurred speech or aphasia, loss of consciousness, weakness or paralysis on one side of the body, headache, and sudden onset of vision disturbances or confusion. A stroke is always a medical emergency that requires immediate intervention as some treatments, such as thrombolytics to dissolve clots, should be initiated within 3 hours.

DIABETIC KETOACIDOSIS

Diabetic ketoacidosis (DKA) is a complication of diabetes mellitus. Inadequate production of insulin results in glucose being unavailable for metabolism, so lipolysis (i.e., breakdown of fat) produces free fatty acids as an alternate fuel source. Glycerol in both fat cells and the liver is converted to ketone bodies, which are used for cellular metabolism less efficiently than glucose. The ketone bodies lower serum pH, leading to ketoacidosis. Symptoms include:

- Kussmaul respirations, which is hyperventilation to eliminate a buildup of carbon dioxide, associated with "ketone breath"
- Fluid imbalance, including loss of potassium and other electrolytes, resulting in dehydration and diuresis with excess thirst
- Cardiac arrhythmias, related to potassium loss, leading to cardiac arrest
- Ketonuria
- Hyperglycemia (elevated glucose); normal values (fasting):
  o Neonate: 40-60 mg/dL
  o Younger than12 months: 50-90 mg/dL
  o Child: 60-100 mg/dL
  o Adult: 65-99 mg/dL or up to 125 mg/dL (diabetics)

Glucose testing should be done immediately if DKA is suspected and a physician notified as treatment with insulin must be initiated.

ACUTE HYPOGLYCEMIA

Acute hypoglycemia (hyperinsulinism) may result from pancreatic islet tumors, hyperplasia, increased insulin production, or the use of insulin to control diabetes mellitus. Hyperinsulinism can cause damage to the central nervous and cardiopulmonary systems, interfering with the functioning of the brain and causing neurological impairment. Too little food, too much insulin, or too much exercise can all trigger hypoglycemia in the diabetic. Symptoms include the following:

- Blood glucose less than 40 mg/dL in neonates and less than 50-60 mg/dL for others.
- Central nervous system: seizures, altered consciousness, lethargy, and poor feeding with vomiting, myoclonus, respiratory distress, diaphoresis, hypothermia, and cyanosis.
- Adrenergic system: diaphoresis, tremor, tachycardia, palpitation, hunger, and anxiety.

Treatment depends on the underlying cause, but glucose/glucagon should be available during the polysomnogram for patients who take insulin and should be administered immediately with signs

60

of hypoglycemia, supported by blood glucose testing. The physician should be notified as other medications may be indicated to increase blood glucose levels.

AIRWAY OBSTRUCTION

With **airway obstruction**, the person usually begins coughing. If the person can respond verbally to the question, "Are you choking?" the airway is not completely obstructed. The patient is encouraged to cough up the foreign body; however, if the person cannot respond, loses consciousness, or becomes cyanotic, intervention is needed.

	Adult	Child	Infant
	Past Puberty	1 y/o- Puberty	Under 1 y/o
Conscious Choking	Abdominal thrusts	Abdominal thrusts	5 back slaps and 5 chest thrusts

1. If the victim becomes unconscious, transfer them to a safe position if not already in one-usually supine on the floor.
2. Begin CPR (there is no need to check a pulse) per AHA standards, beginning with chest compressions.
3. Before giving the first rescue breath, check the mouth to see if there is anything that can be removed and if there is anything obvious, remove it. (Do not do a blind "sweep")
4. Resume CPR. If you have been alone, after about 5 cycles of CPR activate emergency response and then continue with CPR until more rescuers arrive.

AMERICAN HEART ASSOCIATION GUIDELINES FOR CPR

The **American Heart Association guidelines for adult cardiopulmonary resuscitation (CPR) for the trained rescuer:**

1. Establish Responsiveness.
2. Activate the emergency response system and get defibrillator if available.
3. Check <u>carotid</u> pulse (only 10 seconds).
4. If there is no pulse, begin CPR.
5. The trained rescuer will do CPR cycles at a ratio of 30 compressions to 2 breaths, checking rhythm every 5 cycles (about two minutes) and resuming CPR immediately after rhythm check.
6. If the victim is connected to a defibrillator, check the rhythm after 5 cycles (about 2 minutes) of CPR.
7. If the defibrillator indicates shock, give 1 shock and resume CPR immediately for two minutes.
8. Continue CPR and defibrillation until victim starts to move or advanced care can begin.

RACE Guidelines for Fires

In response to a fire, the sleep technician must immediately take action to protect the patient and sound an alarm, and use the **RACE guidelines**.

Rescue	Remove patient from danger.
Alarm	Sound the alarm to alert others, including the fire department.
Contain	Use extinguishers as appropriate (using multipurpose initially if that is all that is available): Class A: For combustibles, such as wood and paper, use water. Class B: For flammable liquids, such as solvents, paints, gasoline, use dry chemical extinguishers. Class C: For electrical equipment, use carbon dioxide and dry-chemical extinguishers. Class A and Class B can be used if the current is turned off. Class D: For combustible metals, such as magnesium, titanium, sodium, potassium, use special dry compound powders.
Evacuate	Exit the area of the fire immediately, and evacuate the entire building if the fire is not completely contained in a very small area (e.g., a waste can) as fire can spread rapidly and unpredictably.

Sleep Physiology Recognition and Summary

Sleep Stages

CLASSIFICATION OF SLEEP STUDIES

Sleep studies are classified as types 1-4, depending upon the montage and place of testing:

- **Type 1:** Nocturnal polysomnograms are completed in a sleep center. Type 1 sleep study must include at least twelve channels of information, including electroencephalogram (EEG), electrocardiogram (ECG), electrooculogram (EOG), electromyogram (EMG, both chin and limb), pulse oximetry, and respiratory effort and airflow sensors. Type 1 is used to diagnose obstructive sleep apnea syndrome (OSAS) as well as other sleep disorders.
- **Types 2, 3, and 4** are modified home sleep studies, using portable devices. These types are appropriate only for OSAS because they provide limited information and are unattended.
  - **Type 2** must include at least seven channels of information: EEG, ECG, EOG, EMG, pulse oximetry, respiratory effort, and airflow sensors.
  - **Type 3** must include at least three channels of information: one ECG lead to monitor heart rate, pulse oximetry, and two sensors for respiratory effort and airflow.
  - **Type 4** must include one to three channels of information, including airflow and respiratory effort sensors.

CORRECT SCORING OF POLYSOMNOGRAMS

Correct scoring of the polysomnogram depends in part on quality assurance efforts. Each epoch must be scored for the stage of sleep, arousals, respiratory events, and limb movements. Computerized scoring may be used but must be quality-controlled and verified. Interscorer reliability testing must be completed with a certified sleep specialist serving as the reference scorer. Interscorer reliability scoring must be done on 200 consecutive epochs (30 seconds) for three or more patients quarterly. There must be agreement in all scoring areas between the reference scorer and other scorers. Every study must include a complete epoch-by-epoch study of all raw data, and the sleep technician must sign to signify that a complete review of the data was completed. The signed form may be kept as part of the patient's record or separately. Interscorer reliability scoring must be done on four portable monitoring recordings (200 epochs for constant analysis of 30-180 seconds) each year for labs that use portable recording devices outside of the facility.

WAKEFULNESS

Wakefulness (stage W) can be characterized by an electroencephalogram (EEG), an electromyogram (EMG), and an electrooculogram (EOG). Scoring is done by epochs, generally a 30-

second record (300 mm), with only one stage of sleep scored for each epoch even though the sleep stage may vary. The epoch is assigned the primary sleep stage.

EEG	Varies according to level of wakefulness: Awake/alert (eyes open): There is low-voltage and high-frequency activity. Relaxed: There is low-amplitude activity. Drowsy (eyes closed): Alpha activity (8-13 cycles/sec) is more than 50% of epoch and is observed most often from the occipital leads but may be present in the central leads or the EOG channel; alpha activity abates if the eyes are open. (For 10-20% of individuals, only limited alpha movement is generated with eye closure.)
EMG	There is usually various high-voltage activity on the chin EMG.
EOG	Varies according to level of wakefulness: Awake/alert: There is frequent blinking. Drowsy: If eyes are closed, movements are slow and rolling. If eyes are open, rapid eye movements are often noted.

SCORING

Stage W (wakefulness) may vary from wide awake and alert to drowsy; alpha rhythms are usually present if the patient's eyes are closed, although about 10% of patients do not exhibit alpha rhythms.

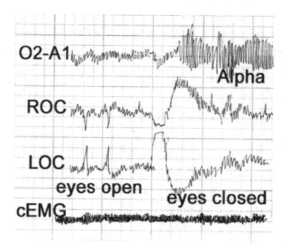

An epoch is scored stage W with these findings:

- About 50% or more of epoch demonstrates alpha rhythm (occipital leads).
- Eye blinks occur with a frequency of 0.5-2 Hz or reading eye movements (slow phase in one direction and rapid phase in the other), or irregular conjugate REMs occur with normal or increased chin electromyogram activity (usually amplitude is higher than during stages of sleep).

STAGE N1

Stage N1 sleep is the transitional period between wakefulness and sleep and may occur with initial onset of sleep or after arousal. In adults, stage N1 sleep occurs in 2%-5% of total sleep time. This stage usually lasts only a few minutes before the patient enters stage N2 sleep. The patient is easily aroused in stage N1. Stage N1 sleep is characterized on the electroencephalogram (EEG), electromyogram (EMG), and electrooculogram (EOG) as follows:

EEG	Alpha activity ceases or decreases to less than 50% of epoch.
	Activity is low amplitude and mixed frequency (2-7 Hz).
	Vertex sharp negative waves (V waves) are over the central scalp area.
	Children and adolescents have high-voltage synchronous bursts of theta activity.
	No sleep spindles or K complexes or 3 minutes or more between episodes are seen.
EMG	High-voltage activity in a chin EMG is similar to or less than during stage W.
EOG	There is some evidence of slow-rolling eye movement, especially at onset, with initial deflection of more than 500 milliseconds.

SCORING

Scoring stage N1 includes alpha waves that attenuate (but only if stage W included alpha waves), and low-amplitude, mixed-frequency activity that occurs for more than 50% of epoch. Stage N1 sleep is generally characterized by slow eye movements, V waves, and low-amplitude, mixed-frequency electroencephalogram (EEG) activity. If stage W does not include alpha waves, then stage N1 sleep is scored with one or more of the following:

- Slowing of EEG background frequencies by 1 Hz or more from stage W with activity ranging from 4-7 Hz.
- V waves.
- Slow eye movements.

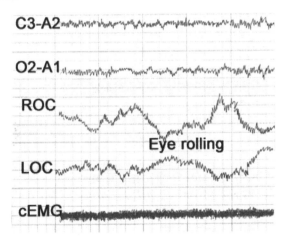

STAGE N2

Stage N2 is characterized on electroencephalogram (EEG), electromyogram (EMG), and electrooculogram (EOG) as described below:

EEG	Activity is low amplitude, mixed frequency.
	K complexes (sharp negative wave preceding slower positive wave, persisting ≥ 0.5 seconds) and sleep spindles (bursts of rhythmic activity 11-16 Hz, persisting for ≥ 0.5 seconds) are evident but may not appear in each epoch.
EMG	Low-voltage muscle activity is shown on a chin EMG.
EOG	Occasional slow-rolling eye movements are observed at onset, but more commonly, there is an absence of movement.

SCORING

Scoring N2 must take into consideration both K complexes and sleep spindles, which characterize this stage of sleep.

- **Beginning:** The appearance of one or more K complexes (not associated with arousal) and one or more sleep spindles signals the beginning.
- **Continuing:** The electroencephalogram (EEG) shows low-amplitude, mixed-frequency activity. Epoch remains stage N2 even without K complexes or sleep spindles if the activity was preceded by a K complex (not associated with arousal) or sleep spindle.
- **Termination:** The end occurs with transition to another stage of sleep, arousal (reverts to stage N1 until the recurrence of a K complex without arousal or sleep spindle), or major body movement with slow eye movements on electrooculogram and low-amplitude, high-frequency EEG activity.

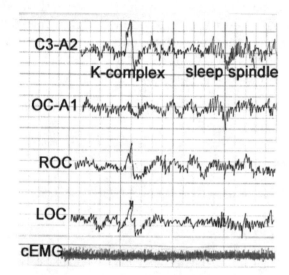

STAGE N3

Stage N3 sleep (formerly stages 3 and 4), also referred to as slow-wave sleep (SWS) or delta sleep, accounts for about 20% of total sleep time for adults. This percentage and amplitude of delta activity is higher for adolescents and lower for older adults. Stage 3 occurs during the first half of sleep. The patient is not easily aroused from stage 3 sleep by external stimuli, such as noise or movement. Parasomnias (e.g., sleep walking, enuresis, night terrors) occur during this stage. Stage N3 sleep is characterized on electroencephalogram (EEG), electromyogram (EMG), and electrooculogram (EOG) as described below:

EEG	Delta activity (> 75 microvolts lasting ≥ 0.5 seconds, 0.5-2 Hz) is evident for 20%-50% or more of epoch.
	Sleep spindles may occur.
EMG	There is lower voltage activity in the chin EMG than in stages N1 or N2.
EOG	There is usually no activity.

SCORING

Scoring stage N3 sleep, also referred to as slow-wave or delta sleep, begins when delta waves occur in 20% or more of an epoch, regardless of age. These slow waves are typically reflected in the electrooculogram channels. Eye movements do not usually occur with stage N3 sleep. Sleep spindles may occur at times. Slow-wave activity is in the frequency of 0.5-2 Hz with an amplitude of

66

>75 microvolts (frontal) and a duration of 0.5 seconds or more. The chin electromyogram usually shows lower amplitude than in stage N2 sleep. Previous staging methods divided stage N3 into stages 3 and 4, stage 3 was scored when delta waves occurred in 20%-50% of an epoch, and stage 4, when they occurred in 50% or more of an epoch.

TRANSITION PERIOD BETWEEN STAGE N2 AND STAGE R

The transition period between stage N2 and stage R is scored, according to the following guidelines:

- **Score stage R** if there is a drop in chin electromyogram (cEMG) tone similar to that found in stage R in the first half of epoch even without REM if there is the absence of **both** non-arousal-associated K complexes and sleep spindles.
- **Score stage R** if there are minimal cEMG tones (but no drop) and **both** the absence of non-arousal-associated K complexes **and** absence of sleep spindles (even without REM).
- **Score stage N2** if there is a drop in cEMG to level of stage R but **both** the presence of non-arousal-associated K complexes or sleep spindles **and** the absence of REM.

STAGE R SLEEP

Stage R sleep, also referred to as REM, has both a tonic stage that occurs without eye movement and a phasic stage with rapid eye movements; it occupies about 25% of total sleep time for adults. Dreaming most often occurs during stage R sleep as well as sexual arousal (penile/clitoral erection). The electrocardiogram may show variations in heart rate, and sensors may indicate differences in respirations related to the phasic stage. Nightmares and sleep behavior disorder occur during stage R sleep. Patients arouse less easily from stage R sleep. Non-REM and REM cycles typically occur about every 1.5-2 hours.

Electroencephalogram	Low-voltage, mixed-frequency activity with sawtooth theta waves are often evident.
	Sleep spindles and K complexes are absent.
Electromyogram	Usually there is no activity because of atonia associated with stage R sleep, although bursts of activity may occur during the phasic stage.
Electrooculogram	There are bursts of rapid conjugate movements during the phasic stage.

SCORING

Scoring stage R sleep begins with rapid eye movements (REM) [< 500 milliseconds], which are often preceded by sawtooth waves on the electroencephalogram (EEG) [2-6 Hz]. Because of the atonia associated with stage R sleep, electromyogram (EMG) activity is low although brief bursts of activity (< 0.25 seconds) may occur. **Onset:** The EEG shows low amplitude with mixed frequency and a low tone on the chin EMG (cEMG). **Continuation:** With or without REM, following one or more episodes of REM, the cEMG continues to show low tone, the EEG remains unchanged, and there is no evidence of K complexes or sleep spindles. **Termination:** One of following occurs: (1) transition to stage W or stage N3; (2) an increase in cEMG tone and criteria for stage N1 are met; (3) arousal occurs followed by stage N1 findings (mixed-frequency EEG and slow eye movement); (4) major body movement is followed by slow eye movement and a low amplitude EEG with mixed frequency and no K complexes or sleep spindles (stage N1); and (5) one or more non-arousal-associated K complexes or sleep spindles in the first half of epoch without REM.

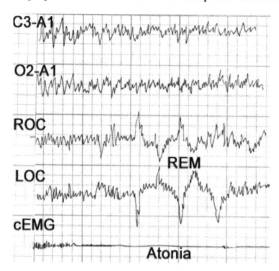

AGE-RELATED FINDINGS IN PEDIATRIC SLEEP SCORING

Pediatric sleep scoring rules apply to children 2 months post-term or older. Because of variations in developmental sleep patterns in pediatric patients, sleep is scored with one additional stage (Stage N). Some findings are age-related.

- Sleep spindles occur at 2-3 months or older.
- K complexes and slow-wave activity (≥ 75 microvolts, 0.5-2 Hz) occur at 4-6 months or older.
- Sleep stages N1, N2, and N3 can be scored in most infants at 5-6 months or older.
- Non-electroencephalographic events can help differentiate sleep in infants 6 months or younger.
  - o REM: chin electromyogram (cEMG) atonia, irregular respirations, REM, and transient muscle activity
  - o NREM: cEMG tone, regular respirations, and no or rare vertical eye movements

DOMINANT POSTERIOR RHYTHM IN PEDIATRIC PATIENTS

The dominant posterior rhythm (DPR) in pediatric patients (infants) is slower over occipital derivations. Electroencephalographic (EEG) readings for infants and children vary, according to age and stage of development.

Age	Findings (Occipital)
3-4 months or younger	Slow, irregular potential changes only
3-4 months (75%)	Irregular amplitude of 50-100 microvolts and a frequency of 3.5-4.5 Hz; attenuates/blocks with eye opening; occurs with passive eye closing
5-6 months up to 12 months (70%)	Amplitude of 50-110 microvolts; a frequency 5-6 Hz
3 years (82%)	Mean frequency of 8 Hz or more (7.5-9.5 Hz)
9 years (65%)	Average amplitude of 50-60 microvolts; mean frequency of 9 Hz; between 6-9 years, 9% with amplitude of 100 microvolts; alpha activity of 30 microvolts or less, rare in children.

Age	Findings (Occipital)
15 years (65%)	Mean frequency of 10 Hz
Adults	Amplitude of 50 microvolts or less; a frequency of 8.5-13 Hz; reactive to eye opening

PEDIATRIC SCORING OF STAGE W

Pediatric scoring of stage W uses the dominant posterior rhythm (DPR) rather than the term alpha rhythm when scoring stage W and stages NREM, using the following criteria:

- Stage W: When 50% or more of epoch has reactive alpha waves or age- appropriate DPR, score stage W.
- Stage W: If there is no reactive alpha waves or age-appropriate DPR, score W with:
  - Eye blinks (vertical eye movements) with a frequency 0.5-2 Hz. Occipital sharp waves occur 100-500 milliseconds after eye blinks and are monophasic or biphasic, 200 microvolts or less, and usually last 200-400 milliseconds.
  - Reading eye movements (e.g., with reading or scanning environment) of a usual duration of 150-250 milliseconds with an amplitude 65 microvolts or less.
  - Irregular conjugate REM and a normal or increased chin electromyogram tone. REM may occur while the child is awake if scanning the environment.

Spontaneous eye closure indicates drowsiness in infants.

PEDIATRIC SLEEP SCORING OF STAGE N

Pediatric Stage N sleep scoring depends on the age of the infant or child. Criteria for staging stage N include the following:

Findings	Scoring
No sleep spindles, K complexes, or high-amplitude, slow-wave activity (0.5-2 Hz) are present in any epoch.	Score as stage N.
Some epochs contain sleep spindles or K complexes, but the remaining epochs have no slow-wave activity for 20% or more of epochs.	Score as stage N2 for epochs with sleep spindles or K complexes and stage N for the rest.
Some epochs contain 20% or more slow-wave activity, and there are no K complexes or sleep spindles in the remaining epochs.	Score as stage N3 for epochs with slow-wave activity and stage N for the rest.
Some epochs contain sleep spindles or K complexes, and slow-wave activity occurs in other epochs.	Do not score as stage N, but score as stage N1, N2, or N3, according to guidelines for older children and adults.

PEDIATRIC SCORING FOR STAGES N1, N2, N3 AND R

Pediatric scoring for stages N1, N2, N3, and R as follows:

Stage N1	With dominant posterior rhythm (DPR), if DPR is attenuated or replaced for more than half of the epoch by low-amplitude, mixed-frequency activity, score as stage N1. Without DPR, score with any of the following: Slowing of 1-2 Hz or more from stage W and activity in 4-7 Hz range Slow eye movements Vertex sharp waves Rhythmic anterior theta activity Hypnagogic hypersynchrony High-amplitude, rhythmic 3-5 Hz activity (diffuse to occipital)
Stage N2	Score as in adults. Sleep spindles usually occur in infants by 4-6 weeks, and K complexes, by 5-6 months.
Stage N3	Score as in adults. Slow-wave activity often ranges from 100-400 microvolts in children.
Stage R	Score as in adults. Activity resembles adults, but frequency increases with age from 3 Hz at 7 weeks, 4-5 Hz (sawtooth) at 5 months, 4-6 Hz at 9 months, and 5-7 Hz (runs and notched thetas) at 1-5 years.

MAJOR BODY MOVEMENTS THAT MAY BE BARRIERS TO SCORING SLEEP STAGES

Major body movements may cause movement and muscle artifacts that obscure readings, sometimes making it impossible to determine the stage of sleep for that particular epoch. An epoch that follows sleep in which 50% or more is obscured by movement is considered movement time. Epochs that include major body movements are scored with the following criteria:

- Score as stage W if alpha rhythm is present for some part of the epoch (even if it is less than 15 seconds in duration).
- Score as stage W without alpha rhythm if the major body movement is preceded or followed by stage W.

If the first two criteria do not apply, score the epoch the same as the epoch that follows the major body movement.

AROUSALS

Arousals are brief sleep disturbances, persisting less than an epoch but interrupting sleep continuity. Arousals indicate fragmented sleep and are associated with daytime drowsiness. Arousals tend to occur more frequently with age. Arousals should be scored, using information from both occipital and central leads. Additional information can be gleaned by observing other electroencephalogram (EEG) channels and respiratory events, but these findings do not alter the basic scoring rules.

- Score arousal for all stages if after 10 or more seconds of stable sleep, there is a sudden change in EEG frequency, including alpha, theta, or frequencies of 16 Hz or more without spindles, persisting for at least 3 seconds.
- During stage R sleep, score arousal if there is an increase in the chin electromyogram at the same time, persisting for 1 second or more.

Stable sleep may begin in a preceding epoch (even one that is a stage W) if it is 10 seconds. All arousals that meet scoring criteria should be scored and used for determining the arousal index.

Respiratory Events

ADJUSTMENTS FOR AIRWAY RESISTANCE AND COMPLIANCE

Airway resistance and compliance are issues that must be considered by the technician when titrating for positive airway pressure because these issues along with patient effort determine the volume of airflow per inspiration.

- If compliance is decreased, which is common in obese patients or those with restrictive pulmonary disease, then higher pressure differences between inspiratory pressure and expiratory pressure are needed to ensure an adequate volume of air during ventilation.
- If compliance is increased, such as from emphysema, then lower pressure differences are needed.
- Increased airway resistance may require higher pressure to deliver an adequate volume of air.
- Increased airway resistance, such as is found in emphysema, often results in prolonged expiration, so the ratio of inspiration to expiration (I:E) may need to be adjusted from the normal 1:2 to 1:4 or more.

SCORING OF APNEAS

Scoring apneas involves scoring from the nadir of the preceding breath to the beginning of the next normal breath, based on baseline respiratory amplitude. If it is difficult to ascertain the baseline amplitude because of respiratory variability, then the apnea is terminated with a marked increase in amplitude, or if there is desaturation, with an increase of 2% in saturation level. **Scoring criteria** include all of the following:

- Thermal sensor drops 90% or more below baseline.
- Duration lasts 10 seconds or more (with at least 90% with reduced amplitude that marks apnea).

The degree of inspiratory effort determines the **classification of apneas** (if they also meet scoring criteria):

- Obstructive: Inspiratory effort continues or increases throughout the apneic period.
- Central: Inspiratory effort is absent during apneic period.
- Mixed: Inspiratory effort is absent for the initial apneic period but resumes during the second half of the apneic period.

SCORING OF HYPOPNEAS

Scoring hypopneas is similar to scoring apneas. The beginning and ending points for hypopnea are scored as apneas, from the nadir of the preceding breath to the beginning of the next normal breath, based on respiratory amplitude, or with a marked increase in respiratory amplitude or an increase of 2% in saturation (if desaturation occurs). Recommended **scoring criteria** include all of the following:

- Nasal pressure (or alternative sensor): Excursions drop ≥30% or more from baseline.
- Duration: The duration of the above drop is ≥10 seconds.
- Oxygen saturation (SpO_2): There is a ≥3% or more desaturation from baseline. (Or the above is associated with arousal)

Alternative acceptable scoring criteria:

- Same first two points from above.
- SpO_2: There is a ≥4% or more desaturation from baseline.

The technologist should note which criteria are used to score hypopneas. The technologist should also note the presence of supplemental oxygen because it may blunt desaturation.

SCORING OF RERA AND HYPOVENTILATION

Respiratory effort-related arousal (RERA) occurs when the airway narrows during sleep, usually indicated by snoring. Although the constricted airway does not result in apnea or hypopnea, it does cause a brief arousal. Criteria for scoring RERA include the following: The sequence of respirations indicates increased respiratory effort or flattening of nasal pressure waveforms with a duration of 10 seconds or more, leading to an arousal from sleep (if not meeting criteria for apnea or hypopnea). Scoring is most effective if done in conjunction with esophageal pressure sensors, although nasal pressure/inductance plethysmography can also be used for scoring.

Hypoventilation is based on PCO_2 scores on awakening and not on persistent desaturation. The use of other sensors is not considered adequate to determine hypoventilation. Criteria include the following: The PCO_2 level (immediately after awakening) increases 10 mmHg or more as compared to the baseline awake/supine value or an increase to a value >55 mmHg for ≥10 minutes.

SCORING OF CHEYNE-STOKES RESPIRATIONS

Cheyne-Stokes respirations are periodic breathing characterized by periods of apnea, alternating with rapid respirations that increase in intensity and then decrease in a crescendo-to-decrescendo pattern. Pulse oximetry shows a wave-like waveform as saturation begins to fall during the apneic period and then rises after the periods of rapid respirations. Cheyne-Stokes breathing is common before death but can also occur with central nervous system damage (e.g., brain tumor, traumatic brain injury, strokes), hyperventilation, and heart failure. **Criteria for scoring Cheyne-Stokes respirations** are BOTH:

- ≥3 consecutive central apneas/hypopneas, which are separated by a crescendo/decrescendo breathing change. Each cycle will be ≥40 seconds.
- ≥5 central apneas or hypopneas/hour of sleep, which are noted over at least a ≥2 hours of monitoring and associated with the hallmark crescendo and decrescendo pattern.

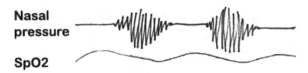

SCORING OF PEDIATRIC APNEAS

Scoring pediatric apneas uses the criteria listed below. This scoring for respiratory events is used for infants and children up to 18 years of age, although some centers may score adolescents 13 years of age or older, using adult criteria, depending on their size and development.

Obstructive sleep apnea (OSA)	All of the following: Duration: Two or more missed respirations (or duration of two respirations based on baseline recordings); duration is measured from end of last preceding normal breath to beginning of next normal breath. Amplitude: There is a 90% or more decrease for 90% or more of events compared to baseline. Inspiratory effort continues or increases throughout the apneic period.
Central sleep apnea	One of the following: Duration is 20 or more seconds. Duration is two or more missed respirations (or equivalent), associated with arousal, awakening, or desaturation of 3% or more.
Mixed sleep apnea	Same as scoring for OSA except inspiratory effort is absent initially but resumes before the apneic event terminates.

SCORING OF PEDIATRIC HYPOPNEAS, PERIODIC BREATHING, AND HYPOVENTILATION

Pediatric hypopneas are scored using nasal pressure sensors, although thermal sensors may be substituted, using the same criteria, if necessary as long as the signal quality is adequate. Respiratory effort-related arousals (RERAs) must be scored with an esophageal sensor. Criteria for scoring pediatric hypopneas include all of the following:

- Peak signal excursions decrease by ≥30% of baseline.
- Duration: The pressure change above is for two or more breaths.
- Arousal, awakening, or 3% or more desaturation occurs.

Periodic breathing criteria include three or more episodes of central apnea, persisting for 3 seconds or more with 20 seconds or less of normal breathing between events.

Hypoventilation criteria include greater than 25% of total sleep time is spent with PCO_2 greater than 50 mmHg (according to transcutaneous PCO_2 or $etCO_2$ sensors).

SCORING OF PEDIATRIC RESPIRATORY EFFORT-RELATED AROUSALS

Pediatric respiratory effort-related arousals (RERAs) must be scored with adequate esophageal or nasal pressure signals. RERAs do not cause apneas or hypopneas but do restrict airways, resulting in arousal. Criteria are based on the type of sensor and must include all of the following:

Nasal pressure	There is a decrease in amplitude from baseline.
	Nasal pressure waveforms flatten.
	There is evidence of snoring, nosing respirations, increased PCO2, or observable increased respiratory effort.
	Duration is two or more respirations (or equivalent duration of two respirations based on baseline recordings).
Esophageal pressure	Inspiratory effort increases during event.
	There is evidence of snoring, nosing respirations, increased PCO2, or observable increased respiratory effort.
	Duration is two or more respirations (or equivalent duration of two respirations based on baseline recordings).

Movements

SCORING OF MOVEMENTS

ALTERNATING LEG MUSCLE ACTIVATION

Alternating leg muscle activation (ALMA) occurs with rapid alternating activation of electromyograms (EMGs) in the lower extremities. ALMA may be associated with periodic leg movements of sleep. An ALMA series requires at least four ALMAs at a minimum frequency of 0.5 Hz and a maximum frequency of 3.0 Hz. Duration usually ranges from 100-500 milliseconds. ALMAs are considered benign, do not require treatment, and are unrelated to sleep disorders.

HYPNAGOGIC FOOT TREMORS

Hypnagogic foot tremors (HFTs) are tremors that occur during sleep onset. HFTs may occur in one or both feet. HFTs are most common in stage W but may continue into stages N1 and N2 sleep. HFTs are scored with a minimum of four EMG bursts in the frequency range of 0.3-4.0 Hz. Duration ranges from 250-1000 milliseconds.

EXCESSIVE FRAGMENTARY MYOCLONUS

Scoring excessive fragmentary myoclonus (EFM), which is twitching movements of the fingers, toes, and mouth that may occur during stage W as well as all stages of sleep, requires that the activity continues for at least 20 minutes of NREM sleep with at least five electromyographic (EMG) potentials per minute. This twitching is similar to that found in REM sleep of normal individuals, but it is more regular. The duration of a burst of activity usually is 150 milliseconds or less, although it may exceed 150 milliseconds if twitching is obvious. Jerking motions are not associated with EFM. In many cases, the twitching is not observable, but activity may be noted on the EMG and the chin EMG. EFM appears to be benign.

BRUXISM

Scoring bruxism, which is grinding of the teeth, is done with masseter electrodes as well as with a chin electromyogram (cEMG). Bruxism may occur with sustained clenching, tonic contractions, or with rhythmic muscle activity, which comprises a series of brief contractions. Some clenching of the teeth is normal during sleep, but excessive grinding of the teeth or jaw clenching may cause damage to the teeth and disrupt sleep. **Requirements for coding bruxism** include the following:

- Phasic (brief) or tonic (sustained) increases in cEMG activity at least two times the amplitude of a background cEMG.
  - o **Phasic**: Sequence of at least three with duration of each 0.25-2 seconds
  - o **Tonic**: Duration of 2 seconds or more
- A new bruxism event is scored only after 3 or more seconds of a stable background cEMG.

Audible scoring: Two or more tooth grinding events a night (in the absence of epilepsy)

REM SLEEP BEHAVIOR DISORDER

Scoring a REM sleep behavior disorder (RBD) requires a polysomnogram (PSG) and a video, audio, or clinical history of REM occurring without atonia or with excessive muscle activity. Some transient muscle activity, usually involving the muscles of the hands, feet, or mouth, often occurs during REM sleep. Some large muscle activity may also occur but does not involve muscle activity across joints. With RBD, a baseline chin electromyogram (cEMG) and an anterior tibialis EMG (atEMG) may have a slightly higher frequency than usually occurs because the state of atonia that normally occurs is missing. **Scoring RBD during REM sleep uses the following criteria:**

- Sustained muscle activity: REM epoch with 50% or more increased cEMG activity.
- Excessive transient muscle activity: 50% or more of ten mini-epochs.
- (3-second intervals in a 30-second epoch); includes bursts of muscle activity, usually 0.1-5.0 seconds in duration with amplitude increased fourfold over baseline EMG activity.

RHYTHMIC MOVEMENT DISORDER

Scoring rhythmic movement disorder (RMD), which is very common in infants, beginning at about 6 months of age and continuing until 2-3 years of age, is dependent on the criteria listed below. The incidence after age 5 is rare unless a patient has an injury to the central nervous system. RMD often includes rocking, head banging, or head rolling, although some children may have leg banging and body rolling as well. RMD most often occurs during stage W when the patient is very drowsy or during stage N1 sleep. These rhythmic movements may be accompanied by humming. **Criteria for scoring RMD** include the following:

- There are clusters of four or more rhythmic movements.
- Amplitude of each burst is double background EMG activity.
- The frequency ranges between a minimum of 0.5 Hz to a maximum of 2.0 Hz.
- A video synchronized with the polysomnogram is required for diagnosis.

PERIODIC LIMB MOVEMENTS OF SLEEP

Periodic limb movements of sleep (PLMS) are scored as events or series:

- **Event:** An event ranges in duration from 0.5-10 seconds with an increased amplitude on electromyogram (EMG) of 8 microvolts or more. Timing of the event begins at the point of an 8-microvolt increase on EMG above the resting EMG and ends with a period lasting 0.5 seconds or more during which the EMG does not increase more than 2 microvolts above the resting EMG.

- **Series:** A series requires four or more leg consecutive movements with the time between movements, ranging from a minimum of 5 seconds to a maximum of 90 seconds. Leg movements involving both legs are counted as one movement if they occur within 5 seconds of each other.

Leg movements are not scored if they occur 0.5 seconds before or 0.5 seconds after an episode of apnea or hypopnea. Leg movements and arousals are considered as associated events if one occurs within 0.5 seconds after the end of the other, regardless of which one occurred first.

Cardiac Events

NORMAL CONDUCTION OF THE HEART

The normal conduction of the heart has four stages:

- Generation of impulse at the sinoatrial (SA) node (primary pacemaker) located at the junction of the right atrium and superior vena cava: The electrical impulse travels in the cells of the atria along internodal pathways, causing electrical stimulation and contraction of the atria.
- Atrioventricular (AV) node conduction of impulse: This occurs when the impulses from the SA node reach the AV node in the right atrial wall near the tricuspid valve. There is a slight delay (about one-tenth of a second), allowing the atria to empty.
- AV bundle (bundle of His) conduction: The AV node relays the impulse to the ventricles through the AV bundle, which are specialized conduction cells in the ventricular septum that branch to the right and left ventricles, carrying the electrical impulse.
- Purkinje fiber conduction: The impulses are conducted down the AV bundles to the base of the heart where they divide into Purkinje fibers, which stimulate the myocardial cells to contract the ventricles.

DETERMINING HEART RATE AND RHYTHM

Determining the heart rate can be done in a number of ways but estimating with a short recording (< 30 seconds) should only be done if cardiac rhythm is essentially regular. The sleep technician should compare 30-second recordings with 6-10-second recordings to determine if there are abnormalities. The normal heart rate varies considerably, ranging from 60-100 beats/min. Methods of counting include the following:

- Count beats for 30-second intervals and multiply x 2.
- Count beats for 14-second intervals and multiply x 4.
- Count the number of R-R intervals in a 6-second reading and multiply by 10.

Heart rhythm should be regular. A normal sinus rhythm is characterized by a P wave and QRS complex present with each beat and having the same appearance:

- P:QRS ratio: 1:1
- P-R interval: 0.12-0.20 seconds
- QRS interval: 0.04-0.11 seconds

SCORING CARDIAC EVENTS

Scoring cardiac events is done with the electrocardiogram (ECG). When evaluating the ECG to determine if arrhythmias are present, the following steps ensure a systematic review, viewing 6- to 10-second recordings:

- Note the absence or presence of P waves: Absence usually means an arrhythmia is not atrial (except with atrial fibrillation or atrial flutter).
- Note the absence, presence, or change in the QRS sequence: Absence indicates AV block or ventricular abnormalities (fibrillation or asystole).
- Note the relationship between the P wave and the QRS complex:
  - P:QRS ratio of 1:1 with more P waves than QRS complexes indicates AV block.
  - P:QRS ratio of less than 1:1 with more QRS complexes than P waves indicates junctional or ventricular arrhythmia.
- Note the P-R and QRS intervals:
  - A shortened P-R interval indicates junctional beat or accessory pathway syndrome.
  - An increased P-R interval indicates AV block.
  - A widened QRS complex indicates bundle branch block (BBB), a beat originating in the ventricles, or aberrant supraventricular beat.
- Note the regularity of rhythm by examining P-P and R-R intervals.
- Note the heart rate.

SINUS BRADYCARDIA

Sinus bradycardia is caused by a decreased rate of impulses from the sinus node. The pulse and electrocardiogram (ECG) usually appear normal except for a slower rate.

Sinus bradycardia is characterized by a slower than normal regular pulse with P waves in front of QRS complexes, which are usually normal in shape and duration. The P-R interval is 0.12-0.20 seconds; the QRS interval is 0.04-0.11 seconds; and the P:QRS ratio is 1:1. Sinus bradycardia may be caused by a number of factors:

- Hypotension and a decrease in oxygenation
- Conditions that lower the body's metabolic needs, such as hypothermia or sleep
- Medications, such as calcium channel blockers and β-blockers
- Vagal stimulation that may result from vomiting, suctioning, or defecating
- Increased intracranial pressure
- Myocardial infarction

Sinus bradycardia is scored during sleep with a sustained heart rate of less than 40 beats/min for patients 6 years of age or more through adulthood.

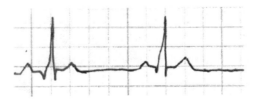

SINUS TACHYCARDIA

Sinus tachycardia occurs when the sinus node impulse increases in frequency. Sinus tachycardia is characterized by a faster than normal regular pulse with P waves before QRS complexes but

77

sometimes a part of a preceding T wave. QRS is usually of normal shape and duration (0.04-0.11 seconds) but may have consistent irregularity. The P-R interval is 0.12-0.20 seconds, and P:QRS ratio is 1:1. The rapid pulse decreases diastolic filling time and causes reduced cardiac output with resultant hypotension. Acute pulmonary edema may result from the decreased ventricular filling if untreated. Sinus tachycardia may be caused by a number of factors:

- Acute blood loss, shock, hypovolemia, and anemia
- Sinus arrhythmia and hypovolemic heart failure
- Hypermetabolic conditions, fever, and infection
- Exertion/exercise and anxiety
- Medications, such as sympathomimetic drugs

Sinus tachycardia is scored during sleep if there is a sustained heart rate of 90 beat/min or more in adults.

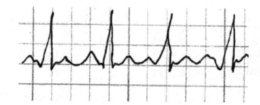

SUPRAVENTRICULAR TACHYCARDIA

Supraventricular tachycardia (> 100 beats/min) may have a sudden onset and result in congestive heart failure. Rates may increase to 200-300 beats/min. Supraventricular tachycardia originates in the atria rather than the ventricles but is controlled by the tissue in the area of the atrioventricular node rather than the sinoatrial node. Rhythm is usually rapid but regular. The P wave is present but may not be clearly defined as it may be obscured by the preceding T wave, and the QRS complex appears normal. The P-R interval is 0.12-0.20 seconds, and the QRS interval is 0.04-0.11 seconds with a P:QRS ratio of 1:1. Supraventricular tachycardia may be episodic with periods of normal heart rate and rhythm between episodes, so it is often referred to as paroxysmal supraventricular tachycardia.

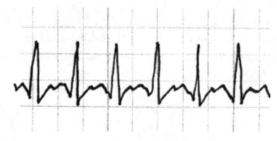

PREMATURE ATRIAL CONTRACTIONS

Premature atrial contractions are essentially extra beats precipitated by an electrical impulse to the atrium before the sinus node impulse. The extra beat may be caused by alcohol, caffeine, nicotine, hypervolemia, hypokalemia, hypermetabolic conditions, atrial ischemia or infarction. Characteristics include an irregular pulse because of extra P waves; the shape and duration of the QRS complex is usually normal (0.04-0.11 seconds) but may be abnormal; the P-R interval remains between 0.12-0.20; and the P:QRS ratio is 1:1. Rhythm is irregular with varying P-P and R-R intervals. Premature atrial contractions can occur in an essentially healthy heart and are not usually cause for concern unless they are frequent (> 6/hr) and cause severe palpitations. In that case, atrial fibrillation should be suspected

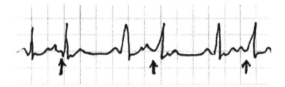

SINUS ARRHYTHMIA

Sinus arrhythmia results from irregular impulses from the sinus node, often paradoxical (increasing with inspiration and decreasing with expiration) because of stimulation of the vagus nerve during inspiration and rarely causes a negative hemodynamic effect. These cyclic changes in the pulse during respiration are quite common in both children and young adults and often lessen with age but may persist in some adults. Sinus arrhythmia can, in some cases, relate to heart or valvular disease and may be increased with vagal stimulation for suctioning, vomiting, or defecating. Sinus arrhythmia is characterized by: a regular pulse of 50-100 beats/min; P waves in front of QRS complexes with a duration of 0.4-0.11 seconds; a shape of the QRS complex that is usually normal; a P-R interval of 0.12-0.20 seconds; and a P:QRS ratio of 1:1.

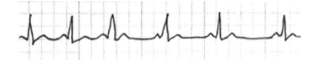

ATRIAL FLUTTER

Atrial flutter occurs when the atrial rate is faster, usually 250-400 beats/min, than the atrioventricular (AV) node conduction rate; thus, not all of the beats are conducted into the ventricles, which are effectively blocked at the AV node, preventing ventricular fibrillation, although some extra ventricular impulses may go though. Atrial flutter is caused by the same conditions that cause atrial fibrillation: coronary artery disease, valvular disease, pulmonary disease, heavy alcohol ingestion, and cardiac surgery. Atrial fibrillation is characterized by atrial rates of 250-400 beats/min with ventricular rates of 75-150 beats/min; ventricular rates are usually regular. P waves are saw-toothed (referred to as F waves); the QRS complex shape and duration of 0.4-0.11 seconds are usually normal; the P-R interval may be hard to calculate because of F waves; and the P:QRS ratio is 2-4:1. Symptoms include chest pain, dyspnea, and hypotension.

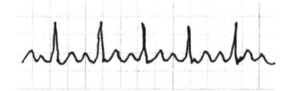

ATRIAL FIBRILLATION

Atrial fibrillation is rapid, disorganized atrial beats that are ineffective in emptying the atria, so that blood pools and can lead to thrombus formation and emboli. The ventricular rate increases with a decreased stroke volume, and cardiac output decreases with increased myocardial ischemia, resulting in palpitations and fatigue. Atrial fibrillation is caused by coronary artery disease, valvular disease, pulmonary disease, heavy alcohol ingestion, and cardiac surgery. Atrial fibrillation is characterized by a very irregular pulse with an atrial rate of 300-600 beats/min and a ventricular rate of 120-200 beats/min; the shape and duration (0.4-0.11 seconds) of the QRS complex is usually normal. Fibrillatory (F) waves are seen instead of P waves. The P-R interval cannot be measured, and the P:QRS ratio is highly variable. This is scored as atrial fibrillation during sleep with irregularly irregular ventricular rhythm and varying rapid oscillations replacing P waves.

SINUS PAUSE

Sinus pause occurs when the sinus node fails to function properly to stimulate heart contractions and the P wave, so there is a pause on the electrocardiogram recording that may persist for a few seconds to minutes, depending on the severity of the dysfunction. A prolonged pause may be difficult to differentiate from cardiac arrest, so the technician should alert medical personnel if the pause persists more than a few seconds. During the sinus pause, the P wave, QRS complex, and the P-R and QRS intervals are all absent. The P:QRS ratio is 1:1, and the rhythm is irregular. The pulse rate may vary widely, usually 60-100 beat/min. Patients frequently complain of dizziness or syncope. Score asystole for pauses of more than 3 seconds for ages 6 through adulthood.

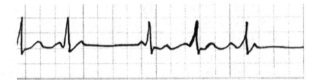

PREMATURE JUNCTIONAL CONTRACTIONS

Premature junctional contractions occur when a premature impulse starts at the atrioventricular (AV) node before the next normal sinus impulse reaches the AV node. The area around the AV node is the junction, and dysrhythmias that arise from that are called junctional dysrhythmias. Premature junctional contractions are similar to premature atrial contractions and generally require no treatment, although they may be an indication of digoxin toxicity. The electrocardiogram may appear basically normal with an early QRS complex that is normal in shape and duration (0.4-0.11 seconds). The P wave may be absent, precede, be part of, or follow the QRS complex with a P-R interval of 0.12 seconds. The P:QRS ratio may vary from less than 1:1 to 1:1 (with an inverted P wave). Rhythm is usually regular at a heart rate of 40-60 beats/min. Significant symptoms related to premature junctional contractions are rare.

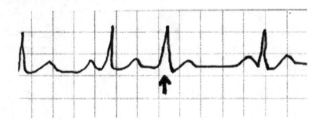

JUNCTIONAL RHYTHMS

Junctional rhythms occur when the atrioventricular (AV) node becomes the pacemaker of the heart because the sinus node is depressed from increased vagal tone, or a block at the AV node prevents sinus node impulses from being transmitted. While the sinus node normally sends impulses of 60-100 beats/min, the AV node junction usually sends impulses at 40-60 beats/min. The QRS complex is of usual shape and duration (0.4-0.11 seconds). The P wave may be inverted and may be absent, hidden, or come after the QRS complex. If the P wave precedes the QRS complex, the P-R interval is less than 0.12 seconds. The P:QRS ratio is less than 1:1 or 1:1. The junctional escape rhythm is a protective mechanism preventing asystole with failure of the sinus node. An accelerated junctional rhythm is similar, but the heart rate is 60-100 beats/min. Junctional tachycardia occurs with a heart rate of over 100 beats/min.

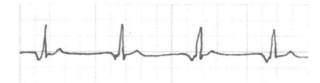

PREMATURE VENTRICULAR CONTRACTIONS

Premature ventricular contractions (PVCs) are those in which the impulse begins in the ventricles and conducts through them before the next sinus impulse. The ectopic QRS complexes may vary in shape, depending on whether there is one site (unifocal), or more (multifocal), that is stimulating the ectopic beats. PVCs usually cause no morbidity unless there is underlying cardiac disease or an acute myocardial infarction. PVCs are characterized by an irregular heart beat; a QRS complex that is 0.12 seconds or more and oddly shaped; a P wave that may be absent or may precede or follow the QRS complex; a P-R interval of less than 0.12 seconds if the P wave is present; and a P:QRS ratio of 0-1:1. Short-term therapy may include lidocaine, but PVCs are often not treated in otherwise healthy people. PVCs may be precipitated by caffeine, nicotine, or alcohol. Because PVCs may occur with any supraventricular dysrhythmia, the underlying rhythm (e.g., atrial fibrillation) must be noted as well as the PVCs.

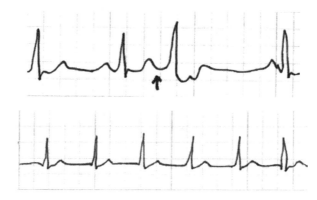

VENTRICULAR TACHYCARDIA

Ventricular tachycardia is three or more premature ventricular contractions (PVCs) in a row with a ventricular rate of 100-200 beats/min. Ventricular tachycardia may be triggered by the same things as PVCs and is often related to underlying coronary artery disease, but the rapid rate of contractions makes ventricular tachycardia dangerous as the ineffective beats may render the person unconscious with no palpable pulse. A detectable rate is usually regular, and the QRS complex is 0.12 seconds or more and abnormally shaped. The P wave may be undetectable with an irregular P-R interval if the P wave is present. The P:QRS ratio is often difficult to ascertain because of the absence of P waves.

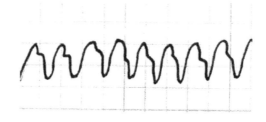

NARROW-COMPLEX AND WIDE-COMPLEX TACHYCARDIAS

For scoring purposes, tachycardias are scored as narrow complex or wide complex. Wide and narrow refer to the configuration of the QRS complex:

- **Wide-complex tachycardia:** About 80% of cases of wide-complex tachycardias are caused by ventricular tachycardia. Wide-complex tachycardia originates at some point below the atrioventricular node and may be associated with palpitations, dyspnea, anxiety, and cardiac arrest. Patients may exhibit diaphoresis. It is scored as a wide-complex tachycardia with three or more consecutive beats at a heart rate of 100 beat/min or more and a QRS complex duration of 0.12 seconds or more.
- **Narrow-complex tachycardia:** Narrow-complex tachycardias are associated with palpitations, dyspnea, and peripheral edema. Narrow-complex tachycardias are generally supraventricular in origin. They are scored as a narrow-complex tachycardia with three or more consecutive beats at a heart rate of 100 beats/min or more and a QRS complex duration of less than 0.12 seconds.

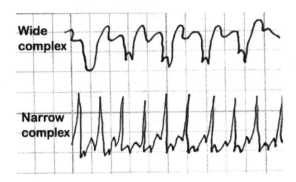

VENTRICULAR FIBRILLATION

Ventricular fibrillation is a rapid, very irregular ventricular rate of more than 300 beats/min with no atrial activity observable on the electrocardiogram (ECG), caused by disorganized electrical activity in the ventricles. The QRS complex is not recognizable as the ECG shows irregular undulations. The causes are the same as for ventricular tachycardia (e.g., alcohol, caffeine, nicotine, underlying coronary disease), and it may result if ventricular tachycardia is not treated. It may also result from an electrical shock or congenital disorder, such as Brugada syndrome. Ventricular fibrillation is accompanied by a lack of a palpable pulse, audible pulse, and respirations and is immediately life-threatening without defibrillation. After emergency defibrillation, the cause should be identified and limited. Mortality is high if ventricular fibrillation occurs as part of a myocardial infarction.

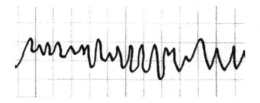

IDIOVENTRICULAR RHYTHMS

Idioventricular rhythm (or ventricular escape rhythm) occurs when the Purkinje fibers below the atrioventricular (AV) node create an impulse. This may occur if the sinus node fails to fire or if there is blockage at the AV node so that the impulse does not go through. Idioventricular rhythm is characterized by a regular ventricular rate of 20-40 beats/min. Rates over 40 beats/min are called accelerated idioventricular rhythm. The P wave is missing, and the QRS complex has a very bizarre and abnormal shape with a duration of 0.12 seconds or more. The low ventricular rate may cause a decrease in cardiac output, often making the patient lose consciousness. In other patients, the idioventricular rhythm may not be associated with reduced cardiac output.

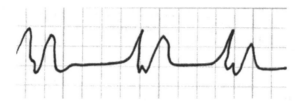

VENTRICULAR ASYSTOLE

Ventricular asystole is the absence of an audible heartbeat, palpable pulse, and respirations, a condition often referred to as "flat-lining" or "cardiac arrest." While the electrocardiogram may show some P waves initially, the QRS complex is absent although there may be an occasional QRS "escape beat." Cardiopulmonary resuscitation is required with intubation for ventilation and establishment of an intravenous line for fluids. Without immediate treatment, the patient will suffer from severe hypoxia and brain death within minutes. Identifying the cause is critical for the patient's survival and could include hypoxia, acidosis, electrolyte imbalance, hypothermia, or drug overdose. Even with immediate treatment, the prognosis is poor, and ventricular asystole is often a sign of impending death.

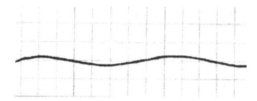

FIRST-DEGREE AV BLOCK

First-degree atrioventricular (AV) block occurs when the atrial impulses are conducted through the AV node to the ventricles at a rate that is slower than normal. While the P wave and the QRS complex are usually normal, the P-R interval is 0.20 seconds or more, and the P:QRS ratio is 1:1. A narrow QRS complex indicates a conduction abnormality only in the AV node, but a widened QRS complex indicates associated damage to the bundle branches as well. Chronic first-degree AV block may be caused by fibrosis or sclerosis of the conduction system related to coronary artery disease, valvular disease, and cardiac myopathies and carries little morbidity. Acute first-degree AV block, on the other hand, is of much more concern and may be related to digoxin toxicity, β-blockers, amiodarone, myocardial infarction, hyperkalemia, or edema related to valvular surgery.

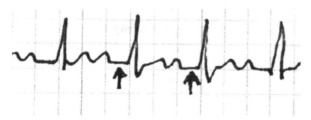

SECOND-DEGREE AV BLOCK

TYPE I

Second-degree atrioventricular (AV) block occurs when some of the atrial beats are blocked. Second-degree AV block is further subdivided, according to patterns of block. With a Mobitz type I block (Wenckebach), each atrial impulse in a group of beats is conducted at a lengthened interval until one fails to conduct (the P-R interval progressively increases), so there are more P waves than QRS complexes, but the QRS complex is usually of normal shape and duration. The sinus node functions at a regular rate, so the P-P interval is regular, but the R-R interval usually shortens with each impulse. The P:QRS ratio varies, such as 3:2, 4:3, and 5:4. This type of block by itself usually does not cause significant morbidity unless associated with inferior wall myocardial infarction.

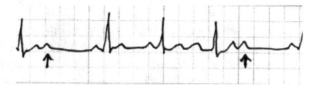

TYPE II AND 2:1 BLOCK

Second-degree atrioventricular (AV) block, type II (Mobitz), is characterized by only some of the atrial impulses conducted unpredictably through the AV node to the ventricles, and the block always occurs below the AV node in the bundle of His, the bundle branches, or the Purkinje fibers. The P-R intervals are the same if impulses are conducted, and the QRS complex is usually widened. The P:QRS ratio varies from 2:1, 3:1, and 4:1. Type II block is more dangerous than type I because it may progress to complete AV block and may produce Stokes-Adams syncope. Additionally, if the block is at the Purkinje fibers, there is no escape impulse. Usually, a transcutaneous cardiac pacemaker and defibrillator should be at the bedside. Symptoms may include chest pain if the heart block is precipitated by myocarditis or myocardial ischemia. With a 2:1 block every other atrial impulse (P:QRS ratio of 2:1) is conducted through the AV node.

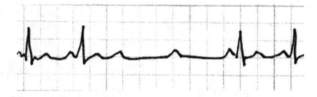

THIRD-DEGREE AV BLOCK

Third-degree atrioventricular (AV) block is characterized by more P waves than QRS complexes with no clear relationship between them and an atrial rate two to three times the pulse rate, so the P-R interval is irregular. If the sinoatrial node malfunctions, the AV node fires at a lower rate, and if the AV node malfunctions, the pacemaker site in the ventricles takes over at a bradycardic rate; thus, with complete AV block, the heart still contracts, but often ineffectually. With this type of block, the atrial P (sinus rhythm or atrial fibrillation) and the ventricular QRS (ventricular escape rhythm) are stimulated by different impulses, so there is AV dissociation. The heart may compensate at rest but cannot keep pace with exertion. The resultant bradycardia may cause congestive heart failure, fainting, or even sudden death, and usually conduction abnormalities slowly worsen. Symptoms include dyspnea, chest pain, and hypotension, which are treated with intravenous atropine. Transcutaneous pacing may be needed. Complete persistent AV block normally requires implanted pacemakers, usually dual chamber.

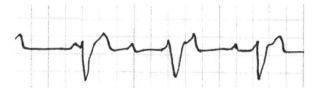

SCORING RBBB AND LBBB

A **right bundle branch block (RBBB)** occurs when conduction is blocked in the right bundle branch that carries impulses from the Bundle of His to the right ventricle. The impulse travels through the left ventricle instead, and then reaches the right ventricle, but this causes a slight delay in contraction of the right ventricle. A RBBB is characterized by normal P waves (as the right atrium still contract appropriately), but the QRS complex is widened and notched (rabbit-eared) in lead V1, which is a reflection of the asynchronous ventricular contraction. The PR interval is normal or prolonged, and the QRS interval is > 0.12 seconds. P: QRS ratio remains 1:1 with regular rhythms.

A **left bundle branch block (LBBB)** occurs when there is a delay in conduction between the left atrium and left ventricle. It is also characterized by normal P waves, but the QRS complex may be widened with a deep S wave and interval of >0.12 seconds (in lead V1). The PR interval may be normal or prolonged. The P:QRS ratio is 1:1 and rhythm is regular.

In Lead V1:

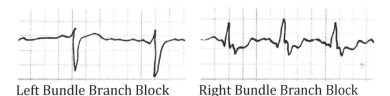

Left Bundle Branch Block   Right Bundle Branch Block

Formulas and Documentation

FORMULAS RELATED TO SLEEP ARCHITECTURE

Apnea-hypopnea index	Number of apneas or hypopneas/hours of sleep (Number of apneas or hypopneas/minutes of sleep) x 60
Desaturation index	Number of desaturation events/hours of sleep (Number of desaturation events/minutes of sleep) x 60
Latency to persistent sleep	Number of epochs from lights out to first epoch of continuous sleep/2 (to provide time in minutes)
Latency to sleep stage	Number of epochs from sleep onset to onset of sleep stage/2 (to provide time in minutes)
Mean duration apnea or hypopnea	Total duration of apneas or hypopneas/number of apneas or hypopneas
Percent movement time	(Minutes of movement time/total sleep time) X 100
Respiratory disturbance index	Number of apneas + number of hypopneas + number of respiratory effort-related arousals (RERAs)/hours of sleep (Number of apneas + number of hypopneas + number of RERAs/minutes of sleep) x 60

Percent sleep efficiency	Total sleep time/total bed time x 100
Sleep onset	First of three consecutive epochs of stage N1 sleep
	Any stage N1 sleep
	Stage N1 sleep contiguous with stage N1 sleep
Sleep period time	Number of epochs/2
Percent sleep stage	(Minutes of sleep stage/total sleep time) X 100
Total recording time	Number of epochs from lights out to lights on/2 (to provide time in minutes)
Total sleep time	Addition of all sleep stages
Total wake time	Wake before sleep + wake after sleep onset + wake after the sleep period

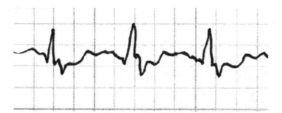

ELEMENTS OF TECHNICIAN SUMMARY DOCUMENTED AFTER SLEEP STUDY

The **documentation** of the results of the sleep study is very important to ensure the appropriate diagnosis is made and the appropriate treatment is prescribed. Documentation is also vital to ensure appropriate insurance reimbursement. The following elements are critical to the documentation of sleep study results:

- The AHI (Apnea-Hypopnea Index) of the patient, which is the average of the number of apnea or hypopnea incidents in each hour of sleep.
- The sleep study must be based on at least 2 hours of recording without a CPAP device.
- A CPAP or BiPAP device can be prescribed if there is an AHI of 15 or more events per hour. In some circumstances, an AHI of 5-14 may qualify a patient for a device if there is also impaired cognition, insomnia, daytime sleepiness, heart disease, or hypertension present.
- The AHI results from the sleep study need to be consistent with the patient's subjective symptoms given when a history is obtained before the test begins. This is the information spoken in the patient's own words regarding how they have felt and what symptoms they have been having.

Therapeutic Treatment and Intervention

CPAP and Bilevel Therapy

EDUCATING PATIENTS ON IMPORTANCE OF SLEEP THERAPY

There are several important benefits of sleep therapy for treating sleep disorders that must be taught to sleep study patients:

- **Feeling more awake during the day:** When the brain gets the rest it needs during deep, uninterrupted sleep, a person feels more alert and focused during the day.
- **Sleeping better at night:** Sleep disorders cause frequent awakenings during the night. When treated, the symptoms of the disorder are controlled, which decreases the number of times a person will wake up during the night.
- **Long-term health benefits:** Untreated sleep disorders are linked to heart disease, hypertension, dysrhythmias, diabetes, stroke, and heart failure.
- **Avoid morning headaches:** A morning headache is a common complaint from patients with a sleep disorder. This is due to dilation of the blood vessels due to increased carbon dioxide levels caused by apneic episodes.
- **Decreased risk of accidents:** Excessive sleepiness during the day can lead to work-related and motor vehicle accidents during the awake hours. According to the National Highway Traffic Safety Administration, drowsy driving causes 2.5% of fatal crashes and 2% of crashes causing injuries.

TESTING REQUIRED BEFORE STARTING PAP THERAPY

Testing with a polysomnogram (PSG) is usually done before positive airway pressure (PAP) is titrated to determine the type of sleep disorder and the need for PAP. This is done in one of two ways:

- **Two-day testing:** The first day of testing involves a nocturnal PSG for diagnosis. If obstructive sleep apnea (OSA) is found, then the patient returns for another night during which continuous PAP titration is completed to determine adequate settings to control apnea.
- **Split-night testing:** This testing uses the first half of the night for a diagnostic PSG. If a clear pattern of OSA is present ($\geq$ 40 apneas-hypopneas in 2 hours or an apnea-hypopnea index of 20-40 with significant oxygen desaturation during this period) or if a diagnosis of OSA has already been made, titration is done in the second half of the night (at least 3 hours). This testing may be used for both the initial diagnosis and follow-up to determine the persistence of symptoms and the effectiveness of treatment.

CONTINUOUS VS. AUTOMATIC AIRWAY PRESSURE

The **differences between continuous (CPAP) and automatic (APAP) airway pressures** have been evaluated by a number of small studies with the following results:

- **Apnea-hypopnea (AHI):** Both CPAP and APAP are equally effective in reducing AHI.
- **Oxygen saturation (SpO_2):** SpO_2 improves with both CPAP and APAP, but APAP is associated with a slightly lower average saturation level.

- **Sleep effectiveness:** Both CPAP and APAP are effective in improving the quality of sleep, including reducing arousals and increasing stage R sleep. Patients requiring high pressures to prevent obstructive sleep apneas (OSAs) usually find sleep quality is better with APAP.
- **Daytime sleepiness (Epworth Sleepiness Score):** APAP and CPAP are generally similar, but some patients, especially those whose OSA is dependent on body position or stage of sleep, rate APAP higher.
- **Airway pressure:** Average airway pressure is lower with APAP than CPAP because of pressure variability.
- **Patient compliance:** Overall compliance is similar with APAP and CPAP.

CPAP

Continuous positive airway pressure (CPAP) can be delivered by a wide range of equipment, starting with the most basic, relatively inexpensive machines to expensive computerized equipment. All positive airway pressure devices have an air blower that delivers pressurized room air to an interface or mask. Pressure can be increased or decreased by adjusting the speed or the amount of airflow, with most machines generating pressure ranging from 2-20 cm H_2O. Carbon dioxide is expelled through a vent or nonrebreather. These may be large or small, but all have filters in the back and can be used with a variety of masks (e.g., oral, nasal, orofacial, nasal pillow). Some have built-in heated humidifiers, and all can be used with cool passover or heated humidifiers. Many basic machines do not adjust for environmental factors, such as altitude, and many do not have an internal memory to generate sleep reports. Some may switch between 110 and 220 volts. Even basic machines allow for a gradual rise to selected pressure. More sophisticated CPAP machines usually have software and downloadable memories that can provide reports regarding respiratory events. Altitude compensation is usually automatic.

DEMONSTRATING PROPER USE PRIOR TO PATIENT USE

Demonstration of continuous positive airway pressure (CPAP) with a nasal mask should be given to patients before titration so that they are comfortable with the equipment and understand how it functions.

- **Two-day testing:** The demonstration can take place on the second day of testing before sleep.
- **Split-night testing:** Usually a presumptive diagnosis of obstructive sleep apnea (OSA) has been made, so the demonstration is done before sleep, anticipating that CPAP titration will occur during the second half of the night.

The **initial demonstration** should include:

- An explanation of the physiological changes during OSA and how they affect oxygen levels and breathing.
- An explanation of the parameters of OSA, which are usually 15 periods of apnea or more, lasting 10 sec/min or more, an arousal demonstration by an electroencephalogram shift ($\geq$ 3 seconds), or a drop in oxygen saturation (SpO_2) by 3%-4%.
- Fitting of the mask, headgear, and straps so that they can be easily and quickly applied during the night.
- Practice wearing the mask with and without air pressure.
- An explanation of the titration process.

EQUIPMENT AND PATIENT PREPARATION

Continuous positive airway pressure (CPAP) titration attempts to find the correct pressure that prevents episodes of apnea when they are most severe, usually when the patient is lying supine during stage R sleep; this position promotes collapse of the upper airway, which worsens with REM-associated atonia.

Equipment preparation	Fill humidifier with fresh distilled water (tap water may erode heating element) to maximum fill line.
	Program the machine with the person's setting or set the pressure dial, depending on the type of machine.
	Check the filter to make sure it is in place and clean.
	Set parameters for the ramp button, low pressure to high, and time to maximum (usually 45 minutes). (This function is usually not used during the initial titration.)
Patient preparation	Fit the mask, headgear, and straps. Release straps on one side only so that the mask can be applied quickly without fitting during the night if titration occurs during split-night testing.
	Provide a demonstration of the mask with and without air (even if patient has had a previous demonstration). Apply electrodes and sensors for polysomnography.

PROBLEM ANTICIPATION BEFORE AND DURING CPAP

Continuous positive airway pressure (CPAP) titration begins with equipment preparation and patient preparation. This includes problem anticipation:

- During the demonstration, ask the patient to open the mouth while receiving positive airway pressure (PAP) so the patient can experience a mouth leak. Keeping the mouth open is usually uncomfortable, making it easier to keep the mouth closed.
- Loosen the mask to break the seal during PAP so the patient can experience an air leak (usually felt as air in the eyes or on the face or heard as a whistling or whooshing sound).
- Demonstrate unsnapping the tube and unfastening leads, and ask the patient to practice so the patient can get up to urinate during the night without removing the mask.
- Tell the patient that she or he may feel somewhat uncomfortable with PAP at first but to just relax and try to breathe normally.
- Reassure the patient that it may take longer than normal to fall asleep ($\geq$ 30 minutes) at first.

ADJUSTING PRESSURE

After the CPAP equipment is set, the patient is prepared, and anticipated problems discussed, continuous positive airway pressure (CPAP) titration begins. Titration procedures may vary somewhat, according to the manufacturer's guidelines and sleep center policies.

TITRATION PROCEDURES:

- Begin CPAP treatment when the patient is ready for sleep.
- Begin with pressure at the lowest setting, usually 5 cm H_2O, and maintain this low pressure until the patient falls asleep.
- Check the polysomnographic tracings, and watch the patient for position and signs of snoring, mouth leaks, or air leaks.

- Increase positive airway pressure 1 cm H_2O at a time at set intervals, usually about every 15 minutes, and observe effects, including changes in oxygen saturation, electroencephalogram, electromyogram, and electrocardiogram.
- Ensure that the patient is supine and in stage R sleep for part of the titration period, or position patient in the supine position for sleep.
- Adjust the pressure up or down as indicated until the optimal level is reached, indicated by the absence of periods of apnea, hypopnea, respiratory effort-related arousals, oxygen desaturation, and other sleep disordered breathing, such as snoring.

INTERMEDIARY DEVICES USED BETWEEN CPAP AND BI-PAP

Two intermediary devices, C-Flex and EPR, between continuous airway pressure (CPAP) and bilevel positive airway pressure (Bi-PAP) may improve compliance because some patients cannot tolerate CPAP because of the pressure during exhalation; this often results in discontinuation of treatments or poor compliance.

- **C-Flex** (by Respironics) is an expiratory pressure relief device and is a modified CPAP machine that has some elements of Bi-PAP. It provides a steady inspiratory pressure but allows patients to select a reduction in pressure during expiration in the range of 1-3 cm H_2O. C-Flex monitors airflow, triggering the short pressure reduction when it detects a change to indicate exhalation. The amount of pressure reduction varies slightly with each breath, depending on airflow.
- **EPR** (by ResMed), another expiratory pressure relief device, provides similar relief of pressure during exhalation but does so by reducing motor speed.

BILEVEL POSITIVE AIRWAY PRESSURE

TYPES

Bilevel positive airway pressure (Bi-PAP, BiPAP ST, auto BiPAP) devices deliver two levels of pressure, which can be preset. Inspiratory positive airway pressure (IPAP) is set at a higher level than expiratory airway pressure (EPAP). This allows for the pressure needed to open the airway during inspiration but reduces pressure to facilitate expiration. Typically, Bi-PAP devices do not compensate for altitude and can be used with humidification. Some have software and downloadable memory to generate reports of sleep events.

Bi-PAP ST (spontaneous-timed) devices have two pressure settings for each breath as well as settings for the number of respirations so that they can trigger inspiration if the respiratory rate falls below a preset level, an important consideration for central sleep apnea and other pulmonary disorders. Settings include a spontaneous mode, which triggers increased pressure after the person attempts to breathe, and a timed mode, which triggers increased pressure to initiate respiration within a preset time.

Auto Bi-PAP (auto-titrating) devices are also available and can vary both IPAP and EPAP automatically as needed to promote adequate ventilation.

INDICATIONS

Indications for bilevel positive airway pressure (Bi-PAP) include the following:

- Continuous positive airway pressure (CPAP) intolerance: If the pressure needed to control obstructive sleep apnea (OSA) is high, the patient may have difficulty with expiration (smothering) and may have air leaks, mouth leaks, and difficulty tolerating treatment. Some patients still have difficulty if expiratory positive airway pressure (EPAP) is set too high. Patients who cannot control OSA with CPAP may achieve control with Bi-PAP.
- Central sleep apnea (CSA): Because the central nervous system is not triggering respirations adequately, CSA does not always respond to CPAP alone. In that case, Bi-PAP ST (spontaneous-timed), which triggers respirations if apnea occurs, is used. Specific indications include all of the following:
- OSA has been ruled out as the primary cause of apnea.
- PAP has not proven effective.
- Oxygen saturation is 88% or less continuously for 5 minutes with the usual fraction of inspired oxygen.
- Bi-PAP (with or without ST) demonstrates clinical improvement.
- Bi-PAP does sometimes trigger CSA if the inspiratory positive airway pressure is set significantly higher than EPAP.

USE FOR COPD AND NMDS

Additional indications for bilevel positive airway pressure (Bi-PAP), also referred to as noninvasive positive pressure ventilation (NPPV), rather than continuous positive airway pressure (CPAP), include the following:

- **Chronic obstructive lung disease (COPD)** - Severe COPD may require Bi-PAP because of an impaired ability to ventilate. Specific indications include all of the following:
- There is a $PaCO_2$ of 52 mm Hg or more (awake and with the usual fraction of inspired oxygen [FIO_2]).
- The oxygen saturation (SpO_2) is 88% or less continuously for 5 minutes at minimum of oxygen at 2 L/min.
- Patient does not have obstructive sleep apnea, and CPAP treatment is not effective or ruled out.
- Bi-PAP ST (spontaneous-timed) may be indicated if initial use of Bi-PAP alone is not adequate to control symptoms.
- **Neuromuscular diseases (NMDs)** - NMDs, such as amyotrophic lateral sclerosis, which are thoracic-restrictive, impair the ability to breathe. Specific indications include:
- The $PaCO_2$ is 45 mm Hg or more during waking hours with a normal FIO2 for that patient.
- The SpO_2 is 88% or less continuously for 5 minutes.
- Maximal inspiratory pressure is 60 cm H_2O or less.
- Forced vital capacity is 50% or less of that expected for a patient with an NMD.

USE FOR HEART FAILURE

Additional indications for bilevel positive airway pressure (Bi-PAP)/noninvasive positive pressure ventilation (NNPV) rather than continuous positive airway pressure include **heart failure (with pulmonary edema)**. Heart failure may seriously impact respirations and sleep. With pulmonary edema, the alveoli become compressed with fluid and collapsed so that oxygen-carbon dioxide exchange is impaired. During inspiration, the alveoli do not fill adequately, and they may completely collapse on expiration. Prolonged heart failure is often associated with weakening of the muscles of respiration. During sleep, when muscle activity is lessened, this can increase the symptoms of heart failure. Bi-PAP/NNPV may be indicated because inspiratory positive airway pressure helps to inflate the alveoli during inspiration, and expiratory positive airway pressure prevents collapse of the alveoli during expiration, promoting better air exchange and decreasing the need for supplementary oxygen. Additionally, as heart failure increases, muscle activity is impaired, so Bi-PAP ST (spontaneous-timed) may be needed to trigger respirations. This use is usually restricted to the hospital rather than at home.

USE FOR OBESITY-HYPERVENTILATION SYNDROME

Additional indications for bilevel positive airway pressure (Bi-PAP)/noninvasive positive pressure ventilation (NNPV) rather than continuous positive airway pressure include **obesity hypoventilation syndrome (OHS)**. OHS occurs when the body mass index is 30 kg/m^2 or more, resulting in impaired respirations, hypoxia, and hypercapnia during sleep. The obesity results in impairment of muscles of inspiration, restricting the thorax and causing hypoventilation, leading to hypercapnia. Most patients develop OHS with obstructive sleep apnea (OSA), characterized by five or more apneas-hypopneas an hour. About 10% of patients with OHS have primarily hypercapnia with an increase of 10 mm Hg during sleep. Medicare guidelines for treatment with Bi-PAP/NNPV rather than CPAP include:

- Evidence of central apnea with a polysomnogram.
- An oxygen saturation of 88% or less, persisting for 5 minutes or more.
- With CPAP failure for OSA but a demonstrated improvement with Bi-PAP.
- Evidence of hypercapnia with OSA: awake PaCO$_2$ of 45 mm Hg or less.

TITRATION

Bilevel positive airway pressure (Bi-PAP) titration begins with the same steps as continuous positive airway pressure (CPAP) titration, including educating the patient, mask fitting and application, and a demonstration with practice. Titration steps include the following:

Set initial pressures	Expiratory positive airway pressure (EPAP): Usually set at 4 cm H$_2$O, but if the patient has had prior CPAP, then the EPAP may be set at the lowest pressure that opened the airway.
	Inspiratory positive airway pressure (IPAP): Usually set at 8 cm H2O or at least 4 cm H2O above EPAP, although some technicians prefer to set the initial IPAP at 2 cm H2O above EPAP.
Evaluate	Response to the initial setting must be evaluated to determine if there is evidence of apnea, snoring, or obstruction. If symptoms are clear, then the initial setting may be adequate.
Control apnea	Apneas are monitored and treated first, so if apneas and oxygen desaturation persist, then both the IPAP and EPAP are increased in 2 cm H$_2$O increments every 5 minutes until apneic episodes stop.
	In some cases, EPAP is increased only for obstructive sleep apneas.

Bilevel positive airway pressure (Bi-PAP) titration, after the initial instructions, demonstrations, initial pressures, evaluating, and controlling apnea, includes:

Control hypopnea	Increase inspiratory positive airway pressure (IPAP) only by 1 cm H$_2$O every 15-30 minutes until the apnea-hypopnea index (AHI) is less than 5 and hypopneas stop.

Control desaturation	If desaturation persists after apneas and hypopneas are eliminated, continue to increase IPAP in 1 cm H_2O increments.
	If desaturation does not respond to increases in IPAP alone, increase both IPAP and expiratory positive airway pressure in 1 cm H2O increments.
	If still no response or indications of excess pressure are evident, then stop the increase and adjust downward as necessary, but consider supplementary oxygen.
Monitor snoring	If apneas and hypopneas are eliminated but snoring or limitations in flow persist, then check for air leaks. If a leak persists, reduce pressure until the leak stops, and then slowly increase pressure again until there are five or fewer apneas-hypopneas an hour.

Final monitoring steps with bilevel positive airway pressure (Bi-PAP) titration, after the optimal inspiratory (IPAP) and expiratory (EPAP) positive airway pressure settings are achieved, include the following:

Observe REM sleep	Evaluate breathing patterns while the patient is in a supine position. If abnormalities occur, then increase IPAP and EPAP 1 cm H_2O until abnormalities stop.
Monitor for excess pressure	If central apneas begin to occur regularly (a sign of excess pressure), decrease IPAP only (maintaining at least a 4-cm H_2O difference between IPAP and EPAP).
	If the difference between IPAP and EPAP is less than 4 cm H2O or there is no response to a decrease in IPAP only, decrease both IPAP and EPAP.
Control central sleep apneas (CSAs)	If CSAs begin to occur before the optimal setting to treat obstructive apnea, use a timed mode for Bi-PAP with backup respiratory rate, and decrease EPAP and IPAP to 2 cm H_2O before the onset of CSAs; then increase IPAP only by 1-2 cm H_2O until there are five or fewer apneas-hypopneas an hour.

CARBON DIOXIDE MONITORING

With bilevel positive airway (Bi-PAP) titration, additional monitoring may be used. **Carbon dioxide** may be monitored as an indirect method to determine $PaCO_2$ and evidence of hypercapnia.

- **PetCO₂:** Exhaled end-tidal carbon dioxide levels, using respiratory spectrometry or infrared spectrophotometry, are not always reliable during sleep so they are rarely used for adults but may be used with pediatric patients to observe for prolonged obstructive hypoventilation (a condition more common to infants and children).
- **PtcCO₂:** Transcutaneous carbon dioxide monitoring, using a silver chloride electrode or infrared capnometer, likewise is used for pediatric polysomnography but is not always given an adequate estimation of $PaCO_2$ for adults.

Considerations when monitoring carbon dioxide:

- If using carbon dioxide monitoring and it is within normal limits, maintain the inspiratory and expiratory positive airway pressures (I:E) differential at 4-6 cm H_2O.
- If hypercapnia occurs, the I:E differential can increase.

<u>TITRATION GRADING</u>

Bilevel positive airway pressure (Bi-PAP) titration should completely eliminate all indications of sleep-associated breathing disorders, such as periods of apnea or hypopnea and arousals, but this goal may not be realistic, depending on the patient's condition and baseline apnea-hypopnea index (AHI) established through initial polysomnography. **Grading of titration adequacy** includes:

- **Excellent**: At least 5 AHI/hr or more and some periods of stage R sleep uninterrupted by arousals
- **Good**: At least 10 AHI/hr or more or by 50% if baseline AHI is 15/hr or less
- **Adequate**: AHI decreased to 75% of baseline although still 10 AHI/hr or more (This is common with severe obstructive sleep apnea syndrome with high rates of AHI.)
- **Inadequate**: AHI more than 75% of baseline and 10-20 AHI/hr or more.

If Bi-PAP is not effective, then the addition of oxygen or more invasive ventilation may be indicated.

TITRATING CPAP AND BI-PAP FOR PEDIATRIC PATIENT POPULATION

Titrating continuous positive airway pressure (CPAP)/bilevel positive airway pressure (Bi-PAP) for pediatric patients should begin with the lowest pressure (generally 4 cm H_2O) with very slow progression because children cannot tolerate the same flow rates as adults and may develop signs of excess pressure, such as increased arousals, using accessory muscles for respiration, decrease in oxygen saturation below baseline, episodes of central apnea, and carbon dioxide retention. Manufacturer's guidelines should be followed closely. The child must be monitored continuously for signs of improvement, such as the elimination of obstructive events, decreased effort of breathing, and adequate airflow. Infants, especially those with Pierre Robin syndrome, characterized by micrognathia with a tongue that causes airflow obstruction, often have more severe obstruction during stage R sleep, and the pressure needed to control symptoms during stage R sleep may disturb sleep during the other sleep stages. Further, even if an infant or child is adequately titrated, requirements may change with development. Infants should be retested about every 3 months initially, extending to every year as their growth stabilizes.

APAP

Automatic positive airway pressure (APAP) devices have self-setting technology to determine the correct pressure for the individual patient and include software and downloadable memory for generation of reports about sleep events. Some machines require specific masks or nasal pillows, and they are not standardized as to settings or the type of reports generated, so the operation manual must be reviewed carefully. These machines are able to detect upper airway obstruction and adjust pressures to compensate. Pressure is adjusted for both inspiration and expiration. Because APAP adjusts automatically, it may be useful during titration in the sleep lab. APAP devices use different sensors, such as vibration sensors to detect snoring and can identify episodes of apnea and hypopnea. APAP devices are set by technicians (according to a physician's prescription) within a range, usually 3-4 cm H_2O and 18-20 cm H_2O.

Adaptive servo-ventilation (ASV) devices provide a baseline positive airway pressure and breathing assist to ensure adequate ventilation (at a preset level) with each breath to 90% of average for the patient.

TITRATION

Automatic positive airway pressure (APAP) titration is sometimes used for the initial positive airway titration. While machines vary, generally they are able to detect upper airway obstruction, limitations in airflow associated with snoring, and apneas-hypopneas, with a variety of different types of built-in sensors. For example, some machines require special masks with vibration sensors that detect snoring. When obstruction occurs that limits airflow, the APAP device increases the pressure until the obstruction resolves. Then, the pressure is slowly reduced until the obstruction recurs, thus determining the correct pressure. Not all APAP devices are able to differentiate between apneas and hypopneas, and some may not identify obstruction not related to snoring. The technician should carefully review data to determine the effectiveness of APAP settings. Additionally, APAP titration levels cannot always be safely applied to continuous positive airway pressure (CPAP), so the effectiveness of the pressure setting with CPAP should be evaluated separately. APAP is contraindicated for congestive heart failure, chronic obstructive pulmonary disease, and obesity-hypoventilation syndrome, central apneas, and previous surgery of upper airway.

Interface Selection

INTERFACES

Interfaces are used with noninvasive ventilation to deliver pressurized air to the patient rather than intubation or tracheostomy. Patients may need to try various interfaces to find one that is effective and comfortable. A number of different types of interfaces are available, all which are secured by straps or headgear.

- **Nasal mask:** This mask fits over the nose but not into the nares. This is useful for patients who are nasal breathers, but the danger of air leaks exists if people breathe through their mouths or are edentulous and if continuous positive airway pressure is high. Risk of aspiration is low because the mouth is free.
- **Oral mask:** This mask fits only over the mouth but is rarely used.
- **Orofacial mask:** The orofacial mask covers the nose and mouth area but usually leaves the eyes free; however, the risk of aspiration is increased. There is more dead space than with a nasal mask, and there is an increased risk of leakage as well as claustrophobia.
- **Nasal pillow:** This mask has "pillows," often made of soft silicone, which fit into each nostril, providing a seal while leaving the bridge of the nose and the mouth exposed. This mask easily dislodges and may dry and irritate nasal passages, but it is less claustrophobic.

NASAL PILLOWS

Nasal pillows are fitted after the patient's nostrils are examined because the pillows that fit into the patient's nostrils are round. If the patient has slot-shaped nostrils, it may be impossible to get an airtight fit, and the pillows may cause pressure and pain. Additionally, some people have different-sized nostrils, so each nostril may need a separate size.

Typically, women use small-to-medium nasal pillows, and men, medium-to-large pillows. Nasal pillows must fit snugly into each nostril because if they are too loose, air will leak. A lubricant (e.g., Ayr) may provide some comfort. Once the pillow size is selected and pillows are attached to the nose piece, the swivel piece is attached, using an angle adapter if necessary; the air hose is positioned midline between the eyes, downward, or to the right or left, depending on the patient's usual sleeping position. The headgear or straps are adjusted to fit. Straps should be snug but not constrictive. One or two fingers should easily slide under the secured strap.

NASAL MASKS

Nasal masks for noninvasive positive pressure ventilation fit over the nose, but the mouth is left free, so nasal masks are not effective for mouth breathers or those who are edentulous. There are many different nasal masks available, so the manufacturer's instructions must be examined before fitting. The piece that fits over the nose is typically soft and made of silicone or a gel material so that it adheres to the skin without causing undue pressure. The nose must be examined to make sure it fits easily into the nasal cup and is not compressed. Any forehead pad must be adjusted so that it is comfortably in the middle of the forehead. The angle between the nose and the forehead is adjusted with the stability adjuster. The headgear and straps are tightened and secured so they fit snuggly while not constricting (allowing one to two fingers to slip beneath straps). The airflow tube is positioned, using the swivel piece, to the most convenient position, depending on the patient's usual sleeping position.

POSSIBLE PROBLEMS

CLAUSTROPHOBIA

Claustrophobia with any interface is common among patients, especially full facemasks, and this anxiety may further impair breathing and cause the patient to feel short of breath. In this case, patients may need time to adjust.

- Ask the patient to practice holding the mask in position without straps or tubing connected, suggesting that the patient read or watch television as a distraction. Encourage patients to pull the mask away from the face if it becomes uncomfortable, deep breathe, and then reposition the mask.
- As the patient becomes more comfortable, follow the same procedure with air flowing through the mask but no straps or headgear. Again, encourage the patient to pull the mask away if it becomes uncomfortable.
- Once the patient can accept airflow, turn off the airflow, attach straps or headgear, and ask the patient to practice wearing the mask while secured. Again, allow the patient to remove the headgear and mask as necessary.
- Last, apply the mask with airflow and headgear in place, but allow the patient to control the duration of treatment until anxiety recedes.
- Allow as many repetitions as necessary.

NOISE

Noise can interfere with sleep by distracting patients and their partners even though the new machines are much quieter than earlier versions. Most people adapt to the noise over time. Patient solutions include:

- Earplugs
- White noise machines
- Soft classical music

For short periods during the daytime, patients can be told to listen to the machine to get used to the sound.

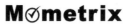

AIR HUNGER

Air hunger is when some patients feel short of breath while using positive airway pressure. Solutions include:

- Examine the mask and tubing for an air leak and correct.
- With ramp pressure, increase beginning pressure as it may be set too low. If using automatic positive air pressure, consult the physician about increasing the starting pressure.
- Use a chinstrap to keep the mouth closed if using a nasal appliance and the mouth is open during sleep, or switch to an orofacial mask.

AIR LEAKS IN FACE MASKS

Air leaks in face masks may occur in spite of the fact that orofacial and nasal masks generally have soft silicone rims that mold to the face; however, if the straps are too tight or the skin is very wrinkled, creases can occur that allow air leaks. Masks often become unseated during the night and leak. Solutions include:

- Reposition the mask by pulling it forward away from the face for 2-3 seconds and then reseat it. Repeat as necessary. This is often sufficient if leaks occur during the night with patient movement.
- Loosen headgear or straps if they are too tight as this can increase the chance of creasing of the skin.
- Apply the mask with airflow turned on as this helps establish a seal.
- Observe the patient carefully during sleep to determine if the airflow tube is positioned correctly for the patient's preferred sleep position as the tube can dislodge the mask.
- Change to a different type or size of interface if leaks persist.

AIR SWALLOWING

Air swallowing can cause burping on awakening and abdominal distention in some patients because some of the pressurized air flows down the esophagus instead of into the lungs. Solutions include:

- Double the pillow under the patient's head to bring the head forward and the chin toward the chest (about a 45° angle) as this position closes off the esophagus. This usually relieves air swallowing for most patients.
- Observe the patient carefully to ensure a change in head position does not impair breathing.
- In some cases, lower pressure settings by small increments and evaluate.

EYE IRRITATION

Eye irritation almost always relates to air leaks and air blowing across the eyes. Solutions include:

- Examine all masks for leaks.
- Reseat or adjust mask fitting as necessary.
- Check straps to make sure they are secure but not too tight.
- Change to a different type or size of mask if other solutions are ineffective.

NASAL IRRITATION

Nasal irritation or dryness sometimes associated with nosebleeds is a common complaint with positive airway pressure, especially with nasal pillows because they are placed inside the nostrils. Solutions include:

- Check the shape and size of the nostrils to ensure that the correct-sized nasal pillows are used for each nostril.
- Use lubricant (e.g., Ayr) during insertion of nasal pillows.
- Increase humidification to reduce dryness.
- Change to a different type of mask if irritation continues.

SKIN IRRITATION

A **rash, skin irritation, or pressure sores** may develop in some patients where the mask contacts the skin or beneath the mask. Solutions include:

- Check the headgear or straps to ensure they are not too tight.
- Instruct the patient to clean the mask each day before use, and observe the patient doing so.
- Make sure the mask is thoroughly dry before applying.
- Provide cushioning protection for pressure sores when applying the mask.
- Refer to a physician for evaluation of possible allergies or the need for medication for a skin rash.
- Consider changing to a different type of mask if other solutions fail.

MOUTH BREATHING AND MOUTH LEAKS

Mouth breathing and **mouth leaks** can exacerbate dryness of the mucous membranes and lead to a reduction in pressure as some of the pressurized air leaks out of the mouth. Additionally, mouth breathing can result in collapse of the upper airways, increasing airway obstruction so that treatment is ineffective for obstructive sleep apnea syndrome. Solutions include:

- Adjust pressure settings and observe for a response.
- Evaluate for nasal congestion or a deviated septum, and refer to a physician for treatment.
- Increase the temperature of heated humidification to relieve nasal irritation and congestion.
- Try a chinstrap to keep the mouth closed (although air can still leak out between the lips).
- Use positive airway pressure with expiratory pressure relief or heated humidifier tubing.
- Change to a full orofacial mask if necessary.
- If the sleeping position is supine, try a supported side-lying position as this may relieve mouth breathing for some patients.
- Do not tape the mouth shut as this can lead to aspiration or asphyxiation.

CHRONIC FATIGUE OR SLEEPINESS

Chronic fatigue or **sleepiness** in patients should show improvement using positive airway pressure (PAP), but sometimes persistent sleepiness occurs despite treatments. Solutions include the following:

- Give the patient time to adjust to the machine as not all patients see results immediately.
- Evaluate the patient's total sleep time (TST) to ensure it is 7 hours a day or more, and ask about daytime napping, which must be included in TST.
- Check the mask for leaks as inadequate pressure may result in apnea and poor sleep quality.
- Review symptoms associated with a poorly fitted mask or mouth breathing, such as dry mouth, sore nasal passages, and dry eyes.

- Review sleep hygiene with patient.
- Discuss habits related to alcohol, caffeine, and cigarettes before bed as these may impair sleeping.
- Evaluate environmental factors, such as temperature, noise, bed partners, or interruptions.
- Ask about restless legs syndrome or bruxism as these may interfere with sleep.
- Observe the patient during sleep to determine if the PAP device remains in place throughout the night.
- Reassess the type of mask used.

Considerations

HUMIDIFIERS THAT MAY BE INTEGRATED INTO PAP THERAPY

Humidifiers may be integrated into the positive airway pressure (PAP) device or external devices connected by tubing. When PAP therapy is delivered without humidification, the flow of pressurized air can exceed the ability of the nose to warm and moisten the air, resulting in drying of mucous membranes. The body compensates by increasing blood supply, resulting in swelling that narrows the airway and increases mouth breathing and mouth leaks. Two types of humidifiers are described below:

- **Cold passover:** The pressurized air passes over a reservoir of water, picking up humidity; however, warm air holds more water than cold air, so the amount of humidification is quite limited; studies show that cold-pass humidification does little to reduce the drying of mucous membranes.
- **Heated:** The water reservoir has a heating element, and the temperature can be adjusted up or down to control the amount of humidification. Pressurized air passes over the warmed water, picking up humidity. Heated humidification can prevent the drying of mucous membranes and relieve congestion, increasing patient comfort and compliance with treatment.

HEATED HUMIDIFIERS

Heated humidifiers increase the amount of water in the pressurized air, but the level of humidification that leaves the machine and that is received by the patient can vary for a variety of reasons:

- **Ambient temperature:** As the air travels through the tubing, the temperature of the air changes, according to ambient temperature, so if temperature falls during the night and cools the tubing and the pressurized air, then the level of humidification also changes.
- **Condensation:** As air cools, its ability to hold water decreases, so condensation begins to form in the tubing, resulting in audible gurgling and decreased pressure, so preventing condensation is critically important for therapy. **Solutions to reduce condensation include:**
  - Increase room temperature 5 or 6 degrees at night or during cold weather.
  - Decrease the level of humidification.
  - Insulate tubing to reduce the effects of ambient temperature.
  - Use heated tubing.

USE OF PAP FOR HOME TITRATION/TREATMENT

Home titration and treatment of sleep disorders have become more common as automatic positive airway pressure (APAP) devices have become readily available and sophisticated;

physicians have begun to send patients who have a presumptive diagnosis of obstructive sleep apnea syndrome home with APAP or continuous positive airway (CPAP) devices to self-titrate and treat, often with minimal instructions and no diagnostic polysomnography. **Considerations** include:

- Patients with CPAP may set pressures to low to be effective or too high, increasing sleeping disorders and sometimes causing central sleep apnea.
- Patients or partners typically use snoring as an indicator of symptom relief, but relieving snoring alone may not resolve apnea-hypopnea issues.
- Diagnosis by guessing is not an effective method of diagnosing sleep disorders, as the presumptive diagnosis may be incorrect.
- Selected patients with APAP may be able to use the machine in the home environment for titrating, but the data should then be reviewed by a sleep technician to determine if the settings are optimal for the patient or if further testing or treatment is indicated.

TRAVEL CONSIDERATIONS FOR PATIENTS USING PAP

Travel considerations for patients using positive airway pressure (PAP), must be discussed as patients frequently need to travel; they should be advised to always carry their PAP equipment with them as symptoms may return after missing even 1 day of treatment.

Transporting equipment	Secure in a carrying case (usually provided).
	If traveling by plane, carry the equipment, and store in the passenger compartment as rough handling or temperature extremes in the luggage storage area may damage equipment.
Power issues	Take voltage convertors and adaptors as needed if traveling overseas.
	Take a power extension cord.
	Provide battery-powered backup if necessary (e.g., for camping).
Humidifier	Carry distilled water, or purchase on arrival.
	Compensate for lack of a humidifier with a saline nasal spray or water-soluble gel.
Altitude adjustments	Check altitude and manufacturer's guidelines for adjusting pressure.

ADVERSE EFFECTS OF PAP THERAPY

Positive airway pressure (PAP) therapy can cause a number of **adverse effects,** some because of the equipment but others because of pressure settings or social issues. Compliance (using for 4 hours or more a night 70% or more of the time) depends on identifying adverse effects and helping the patient to find solutions:

- **Nasal irritation** (If PAP is inadequately humidified)
  - Dryness and congestion
  - Watery discharge
  - Bleeding
- **Excess pressure**
  - Air leaks and mouth leaks
  - Air swallowing and difficulty exhaling
  - Discomfort in chest

- o Conjunctivitis (related to air leaks)
- o Increased arousals and difficulty sleeping
- o Barotrauma (lung damage): rare and usually related to blockage of exhalation valve with no pressure release valve or airway pressure alarm; sometimes results in pneumothorax or pneumoencephaly
- **Mask**
  - o Skin irritation
  - o Rash
  - o Ulcerations (usually related to excess pressure or improperly sized mask)
  - o Allergic reaction
- **Social reactions**
  - o Partner conflict
  - o Inconvenience
  - o Resistance to treatment

THERAPIES FOR OBSTRUCTIVE SLEEP APNEA

Potential therapies for obstructive sleep apnea (OSA) include the following:

Continuous positive airway pressure (CPAP)	Education regarding the CPAP devices should include the different types of masks and machines available.
	Bi-level positive airway pressure changes pressure during exhalation to facilitate breathing.
	Auto positive airway pressure has adjustable rather than fixed pressure.
	The technician should explain the importance of using a humidifier to prevent the drying of mucous membranes, and the patient should understand that using CPAP is not a temporary or part-time solution but should be used with every sleep, whether at night or napping during the day.
Oral/dental devices	Some patients with mild OSA may be prescribed oral or dental devices, which fit inside the mouth or are fastened around the head to open the airway during sleep. The most common types of devices are mandibular repositioning and tongue retaining devices.
	Patients should be cautioned to have devices fitted by professionals, such as a dentist, to avoid damage to the teeth, mouth, or jaw.

CPAP FOR OBSTRUCTIVE SLEEP APNEA IN PEDIATRIC PATIENTS

Continuous positive airway pressure (CPAP) is used for obstructive sleep apnea (OSA) in pediatric patients, which may resolve as they grow; however, some children progress to adult

OSA, especially if they were not diagnosed and treated as children. Issues relevant to children include the following:

- Infants younger than 9 months may be started on CPAP immediately without prior practice or behavioral training.
- Tolerance to the interface and treatment varies widely, according to age and temperament. Many children benefit from a staged approach in which they first have polysomnography for diagnosis and are sent home with a nasal mask (hose detached) to practice wearing and adjusting to the mask before they return to the sleep center for titration.
- Fitting the mask can be challenging, and in some cases, specially molded masks to fit the child may be required. Trying a variety of interfaces may help to find one that is effective.
- Warming the tubing or using warm humidification may relieve nasal swelling and discomfort.

USE OF OXYGEN/PAP FOR PULMONARY CHEST DISORDERS AND CARDIAC ABNORMALITIES FOR PEDIATRIC PATIENTS

Pediatric patients with pulmonary disorders (congenital or acquired abnormalities), chest wall deformities, or cardiac abnormalities may require supplementary oxygen with or without positive airway pressure. Oxygen saturation levels (baseline and during Stage R sleep) should be evaluated before titration to ensure that supplementary oxygen is necessary. Oxygen should be administered using the same type of supply that will be available in the home, often a concentrator, beginning with a very low flow. If the child is already receiving oxygen, this flow rate is used initially with **slow increments**:

- Infants: Increments of 0.25 L/min
- Children: Increments of 0.5-1 L/min

Children should be observed carefully for signs of hypoventilation related to decreased hypoxic drive (common in infants and children), so carbon dioxide must be monitored. Titration must include at least one period of stage R sleep as requirements may vary from those of the other sleep stages. The age of the child and the diagnosis are important in determining how frequently the child should be reassessed.

USE OF OXYGEN/PAP FOR HYPOVENTILATION DISORDERS IN PEDIATRIC PATIENTS

Hypoventilation disorders in pediatric patients may require noninvasive ventilation (NIV)/positive airway pressure (PAP) with or without controlled respirations. Hypoventilation may relate to the following:

- **Central nervous system** (e.g., brain injury, Arnold-Chiari malformation): Hypoventilation is most obvious during slow-wave sleep when respirations are primarily under the control of the autonomic nervous system.
- **Obstructive**: This may relate to congenital malformations or obesity.
- **Peripheral**: Muscles of respiration cannot perform adequately.

Nocturnal hypoventilation generally occurs before onset of hypoventilation in wake time. Titration usually begins with PAP only, but humidification and volume control may be indicated for some children. Spontaneous control of respirations is titrated first, followed by a minimal synchronized intermittent mandatory ventilation rate if necessary. End expiratory pressure is increased to promote oxygenation, and the peak pressure or respiratory rate increased for carbon dioxide retention. Children with respiratory failure and progressive neuromuscular disorders may need NIV/PAP or other ventilatory support during the daytime as well as during the night.

EVALUATION OF EFFECTS OF POSITIVE AIRWAY PRESSURE

Effects of positive airway pressure on sleep must be evaluated.

REM latency	REM latency	This is the time period from the first epoch of sleep until the onset of REM sleep.
Sleep efficiency	SE	SE is calculated by comparing the percentage of time spent sleeping to the time spent in bed. If a person sleeps 4 hours and spends 8 hours in bed, the ratio is 4:8, and the SE is 50%. Formula: Total sleep time X 100/total sleep period.
Sleep onset latency	SOL	SOL determines the amount of time needed to go from an awake state to a sleep state. SOL is used with the multiple latency sleep test to judge the severity of sleepiness during the day: 0 − 5 minutes = severe 5 − 10 minutes = moderate 10 − 15 minutes = mild 15 − 20 minutes = normal SOL is also monitored during nocturnal polysomnography, with normal SOL about 10-15 minutes.
Sleep period time	SPT	The SPT is calculated as the percentage of total time spent at different sleep stages. Thus, if 22% of sleep time was spent in REM sleep, the report would read "REM, 22% SPT."
Total sleep time	TST	TST is total sleep in minutes for all stages of sleep (stage 1, 2, and 3 non-REM and REM).
Total sleep period	TSP	TSP begins with lights out and ends with lights on and is calculated in hours and minutes. (sometimes referred to as total bedtime time or TBT).
Total wake time	TWT	TWT is the total number of minutes awake in the TSP (lights out to lights on).
Wake-after-sleep onset	WASO	WASO is the total minutes spent awake after first falling asleep and until the final awakening time.

Oxygen Therapy

COMPRESSED OXYGEN

Oxygen can be supplied in a variety of different forms.

Compressed oxygen	Tanks of compressed oxygen are typically color-coded as white or green, although contents always need to be verified by checking the label on the tank. Tanks are labeled USP and Oxygen in a yellow diamond. Typical sizes include the following: H tanks, which are tall tanks (about 4.5 feet) E tanks, which are small portable tanks for short duration use

	Oxygen is under pressure, so tanks require a regulator, which includes the following: Cylinder valve, which turns the flow of oxygen on or off Pressure reducing valve, which reduces cylinder pressure (2200 psi) to 50 psi Flowmeter (with humidifier), which controls the liter per minute flow of oxygen to the patient. The flowmeter is usually directly attached to a bubble jet humidifier to humidify the oxygen.

LIQUID OXYGEN

Oxygen can be supplied in a variety of different forms.

Liquid oxygen	Liquid oxygen (LOX) is stored at temperatures of -183°C in special cryogenic containers with 1 cubic foot of liquid oxygen equal to 860 cubic feet of oxygen gas. Small 4-pound tanks can be attached to a belt about a person's waist and may last up to 8 hours. One problem is that as the tanks slowly warm, the oxygen evaporates, losing as much as half a liter overnight. LOX is maintained at 21 psi, and tanks continuously vent, so they should be used in well-ventilated areas. Small tanks are usually refilled from a larger liquid oxygen reservoir tank, but touching the fill valve can result in burns. The weight of the tank is used to estimate the amount of oxygen remaining rather than pressure, so it is more difficult to determine the amount remaining.

CONCENTRATED OXYGEN

Oxygen can be supplied in a variety of different forms.

Concentrated oxygen	Concentrators are portable electric devices that filter ambient air to produce oxygen. They are useful only for low-flow oxygen (usually 1-6 L/min) at lower concentrations (ranging from 50%-95%) although some larger devices are able to provide 10 L/min. Concentrators are frequently used for people who need at-home oxygen because they are relatively inexpensive compared to compressed or liquid oxygen. Concentrators are adequate for people who need supplemental rather than pure oxygen, such as those with sleep apnea. Small portable units that can be battery-powered are also available. Concentrators may be used in some sleep centers as well if a central oxygen supply is not available.

HIGH- AND LOW-FLOW OXYGEN DELIVERY DEVICES

High-flow oxygen delivery devices provide oxygen at flow rates higher than the patient's inspiratory flow rate at specific medium-to-high fraction of inspired oxygen (FIO_2), up to 100%. However a flow of 100% oxygen actually provides only 60%-80% FIO_2 to the patient because the patient also breathes in some room air, diluting the oxygen. The actual amount of oxygen received depends on the type of interface or mask. Additionally, the flow rate is actually less than the inspiratory flow rate upon actual delivery. High-flow oxygen delivery is usually not used in the sleep center. Humidification is usually required because the high flow is drying.

Low-flow oxygen delivery devices provide 100% oxygen at flow rates lower than the patient's inspiratory flow rate, but the oxygen mixes with room air, so the FIO_2 varies. Humidification is usually only required if the flow rate is 3 L/min or more. Much oxygen is wasted with exhalation, so

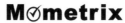

a number of different devices to conserve oxygen are available. Interfaces include transtracheal catheters and cannulae with reservoirs.

OXYGEN INTERFACES

Oxygen interfaces are used for the delivery of oxygen to the patient.

Nasal prongs (cannulae)	This is the most common delivery system for oxygen because of ease of use, providing the fraction of inspired oxygen (FIO_2) of 24%-40% with flows at 6 L/min or less (although the maximum for infants is 2 L/min). Humidification is needed for flow rates of 4 L/min or more.
Oxygen mask	This covers the nose and mouth, delivering FIO_2 of 30%-60%, but the flow of oxygen should be maintained between 6-12 L/min to prevent rebreathing. Because of the higher flow rate, humidification should be used. Oxygen masks are usually used short-term when higher rates of oxygen are needed.
Venturi mask	Oxygen entrainment masks come with different size color-coded nozzles to control the FIO_2 accurately, with different sizes providing different FIO_2 rates, usually ranging from 24%-50%, although a FIO_2 of 35% or more is not always reliable. Flow rate is 12-15 L/min. Air-entrainment humidifiers may be used to add humidification. Oxygen entrainment masks are often used with patients who have chronic obstructive pulmonary disease.

SUPPLEMENTARY OXYGEN AND CENTRAL SLEEP APNEA

Supplementary oxygen may be used with positive airway pressure to treat **central sleep apnea (CSA)** not related to hypercapnia. The oxygen reduces hypoxemia, in turn, reducing reflex hyperventilation and hypocapnia to maintain the arterial carbon dioxide at an adequate level to prevent apnea in some patients. However, if the CSA is hypercapnic, oxygen therapy may cause worsening of the condition, so blood gases must be monitored. Oxygen is titrated during polysomnography until CSA resolves. In some cases, such as with heart disease, medications that improve circulation and oxygenation may relieve CSA. Others may receive stimulant medication rather than oxygen. CSA is most common in adults and premature infants. An infant with CSA is fitted with apnea alarms, which usually waken the infant and trigger respirations.

SUPPLEMENTAL LOW-FLOW OXYGEN

Supplemental low-flow oxygen is used with a polysomnogram, the use of which must be explained by the technician. The appropriate oxygen delivery device should be in place, ensuring that the oxygen will not interfere with airflow measurements. Steps to oxygen titration include:

Initiate	Initiate low-flow supplemental oxygen at 1 L/min when oxygen saturation (SpO_2) falls below 85% on ambient room air.
Monitor	Monitor SpO_2 carefully to ensure it increases to at least 90%. Alternate monitoring methods include obtaining arterial blood gases from indwelling arterial lines and measuring transcutaneous PO_2.
Titrate	Titrate oxygen by slowly increasing the flow rate by 0.5 L/min at a time until the SpO_2 is 90% or more, but do not exceed 4 L/min without a specific physician's order. If higher levels of oxygen are needed, then different oxygen delivery devices may be indicated along with humidification.

Elements of Oxygen Administration

Terms related to **oxygen administration** include:

Flow rate (FR)	The FR is the number of liters of oxygen flow per minute. During titration, flow may be adjusted according to the patient's response, using the least amount required to obtain optimal oxygen saturation. Physicians should set the limit of allowable desaturation before polysomnography.
Fraction of inspired oxygen (FIO_2)	The FIO_2 is the percentage of oxygen in the mixture of air provided the patient. This ranges from that of room air, 21%-100%, but is usually maintained at 60% or less. FIO_2 may be expressed as a decimal or percentage: 0.50 equals 50%. When ordering oxygen for titration, the physician usually does not specify the exact FIO_2 but rather the target oxygen saturation.
Room air (RA)	RA is 21% oxygen. This is the usual air provided by positive airway pressure.

Oxygen Administration During Polysomnography

Oxygen administration during polysomnography follows a protocol of continuous positive airway pressure (CPAP)/bilevel positive airway pressure (Bi-PAP) titration so reports are consistent. Procedures include the following:

- Ensure oxygen does not interfere with airflow sensors. Do not use two sets of nasal prongs, but rather use bifurcated dual tubes that allow for oxygen administration on one side and airflow measurements on the other; however, check to ensure that both nostrils are equal in size and patent.
- Alternately, replace the nasal pressure cannula that measures airflow with the oxygen nasal prongs, and measure directly from the oxygen tubing.
- During CPAP/Bi-PAP titration, the administration of oxygen depends on the type of interface and equipment. Check the manufacturer's guidelines for the addition of oxygen, which may be administered through an oxygen inlet nipple provided or through additional tubing and an adaptor between the humidifier and the patient.
- Keep the flow of oxygen as far away from the electrical equipment as possible.

Safety Precautions for Use of Oxygen

Safety precautions for use of oxygen include the following:

- Avoid using combustible materials (e.g., oils, lotions, sprays) in the presence of oxygen, including collodion.
- Prohibit smoking, matches, or other flame-producing devices near oxygen.
- Secure tanks in an upright position to prevent their falling as the oxygen is under high pressure and the tanks have the potential to explode. They should be stored away from sources of heat.
- Avoid touching liquid oxygen or fill valves as liquid oxygen can burn the tissue severely. Ensure that venting is directed away from the body.
- Use only in well-ventilated areas to decrease the danger of fire.
- Maintain a distance of 6 feet or more between the source of oxygen and electrical equipment, which should be properly grounded.
- Ensure equipment is properly maintained.

OXYGEN TROUBLESHOOTING

Oxygen troubleshooting includes the following:

- If supplemental oxygen does not increase the oxygen saturation (SpO_2), this may indicate that there is a leak in the system that is interfering with oxygen delivery or that monitoring devices, such as the airflow sensor and pulse oximeter are not recording properly, so the technician should examine these.
- The patient should be observed for mouth leaks or mouth breathing that prevents adequate intake of oxygen.
- If measurements are accurate and no problem is found with leaks, then the other equipment, such as the flowmeter and tubing should be checked for functioning and patency.
- If the SpO_2 remains dangerously low, then the technician may need to interrupt the polysomnogram and awaken the patient to ensure that a medical emergency has not occurred.
- If the patient experiences persistent low SpO_2, hypoxia, and respiratory distress on awakening or is unresponsive, the technician should contact the physician.

CPSGT Practice Test #1

1. Twitching movements of the fingers, toes, and mouth that may occur during stage W, non-REM, and REM sleep are known as

    a. bruxism.
    b. excessive fragmentary myoclonus (EFM).
    c. REM sleep behavior disorder (RBD).
    d. rhythmic movement disorder (RMD).

2. The cEMG provides information on all of the following EXCEPT

    a. snoring.
    b. teeth grinding.
    c. electrical activity within the brain.
    d. muscle tone of the chin muscles.

3. Which of the following constitutes good sleep hygiene?

    a. Drinking alcohol before going to bed.
    b. Watching TV in bed right before trying to go to sleep.
    c. Getting up to do something relaxing after 20 minutes in bed without falling asleep.
    d. Taking naps during the day.

4. Which of the following brain structures is involved in autonomic functions, homeostasis, endocrine processes, emotions, and the regulation of sleep?

    a. Hypothalamus.
    b. Mamillary bodies.
    c. Hippocampus.
    d. Posterior pituitary gland.

5. Morning/evening questionnaires ask the patient to indicate which of the following?

    a. How the patient feels in the morning after going to sleep at 9 PM.
    b. The five consecutive hours during the day that the patient would prefer to work.
    c. The patient's appetite two hours after awakening.
    d. All of the above.

6. One criterion for scoring pediatric obstructive sleep apnea is that, compared to baseline, there is a 90% or greater decrease in amplitude for at least what percentage of events?

    a. 25%.
    b. 50%.
    c. 80%.
    d. 90%.

7. Sudden, involuntary, abnormal electrical disturbances in the brain that can manifest as alterations/loss of consciousness and convulsions are known as

    a. generalized tonic-clonic seizures.
    b. primary generalized myoclonic epilepsy.
    c. amyotrophic lateral sclerosis.
    d. West syndrome.

8. What is the range of normal scores on the Fatigue Severity Scale?

   a. 5-15.
   b. 5-20.
   c. 9-25.
   d. 9-35.

9. Which of the following is NOT part of scoring pediatric obstructive sleep apneas?

   a. A duration of two or more missed respirations (or duration of two respirations based on baseline recordings).
   b. Inspiratory effort that continues or increases throughout the apneic period.
   c. Missed respirations associated with arousal, awakening, or desaturation of 3% or more.
   d. A 90% or more decrease in amplitude for 90% or more of events, compared to baseline.

10. Which type of waves have a frequency of 13–35 Hz, an amplitude of less than 30 µV, and are present during normal wakefulness when the patient is alert?

   a. Delta waves.
   b. Beta waves.
   c. Vertex waves.
   d. Theta waves.

11. During polysomnography, which of the following can be caused by skin irritation, such as a rash?

   a. High-frequency artifacts.
   b. Spike in EEG.
   c. High impedance. ·
   d. Slow waves.

12. Pulse oximetry measures

   a. arterial oxygen saturation (SpO_2).
   b. electrical activity in the leg muscles.
   c. venous oxygen saturation.
   d. the degree and duration of snoring.

13. When periodic limb movements of sleep are scored as events, which of the following is FALSE?

   a. An event ranges in duration from 0.5–10 seconds, with an EMG amplitude of 8 µV or more.
   b. Timing of the event begins at the point of an 8-µV increase on EMG.
   c. Timing of the event ends with a period, lasting 0.5 seconds or longer, during which EMG does not rise more than 2 µV.
   d. An event requires four or more consecutive leg movements, with the interval between movements ranging from 5-90 seconds.

14. Which of the following is NOT a way to decrease the amount of condensation in humidifier tubing?

   a. Using heated tubing.
   b. Reducing the level of humidification.
   c. Insulating the tubing.
   d. Decreasing room temperature at night.

15. Which of the following is FALSE with regard to liquid oxygen?

    a. It is stored at -183°C in special cryogenic containers.

    b. It is maintained at 18 psi.

    c. As the tanks slowly warm, the oxygen evaporates.

    d. Touching the fill valve can result in burns.

16. What is the minimum number of hours that an overnight nocturnal polysomnogram (PSG) should last in order to obtain adequate data?

    a. Three.

    b. Four.

    c. Five.

    d. Six.

17. Which of the following is FALSE with regard to the multiple sleep latency test (MSLT)?

    a. Smoking is not allowed within 30 minutes of starting a nap.

    b. Physiological calibrations are done five minutes prior to the onset of the nap period.

    c. A patient should discontinue the use of stimulants two weeks prior to the MSLT.

    d. The MSLT includes seven nap periods.

18. Which of the following is true of supraventricular tachycardia?

    a. It originates in the ventricles.

    b. There may be periods of normal heart rate and rhythm between episodes.

    c. The QRS complex appears abnormal.

    d. The P wave is absent.

19. Which of the following is NOT true of EEG during stage 2 non-REM sleep?

    a. There are periods between K complexes or sleep spindles of less than three minutes that are unrelated to arousal.

    b. Delta activity is less than 20% of the epoch.

    c. Abrupt K-complex clusters and delta waves may indicate arousal.

    d. Activity is high voltage.

20. Which of the following is FALSE with regard to oronasal masks?

    a. There is a greater chance of leakage than with nasal masks.

    b. They cover both the nose and the mouth.

    c. Nasal pillows must fit snugly into each nostril when using this mask.

    d. The masks are often less comfortable for the patient than nasal masks.

21. One criterion for scoring pediatric respiratory effort-related arousals (RERAs) is that nasal pressure is reduced by what percentage, compared to baseline?

    a. 10%.

    b. 15%.

    c. 50%.

    d. 90%.

22. What is the normal range of oxygen saturation?

    a. 85-90%.
    b. 91-94%.
    c. 95-98%.
    d. 99-100%.

23. Which of the following is true of Cheyne-Stokes respirations?

    a. Cheyne-Stokes breathing can occur with damage to the central nervous system (e.g., brain tumor, stroke, traumatic brain injury), hyperventilation, and heart failure.
    b. Pulse oximetry during the respirations shows a wave-like waveform as saturation begins to rise during the apneic period and then falls after the periods of rapid respirations.
    c. One criterion for scoring the respirations is the presence of consecutive cycles of a crescendo-to-decrescendo breathing pattern that lasts for a minimum of two consecutive minutes.
    d. One criterion for scoring the respirations is the presence of consecutive cycles of a crescendo-to-decrescendo breathing pattern that includes three central apneas or central hypopneas per hour of sleep.

24. What is the total daily sleep requirement (including both nighttime sleep and daytime naps) for a two-year-old infant?

    a. 9.5 hours.
    b. 10.25 hours.
    c. 11 hours.
    d. 13 hours.

25. Which of the following is NOT a therapeutic intervention for narcolepsy?

    a. Selective serotonin reuptake inhibitors (SSRIs).
    b. Methylphenidate.
    c. Tricyclic antidepressants (TCAs).
    d. Diet and exercise.

26. Which of the following actions by the sleep technician violates the principles of proper body mechanics?

    a. Avoiding pushing with the arms.
    b. Avoiding twisting to lift.
    c. Using a step stool to reach items.
    d. Bending at the waist to reach items.

27. Which of the following neurotransmitters is increased during the awake state; decreased during stages 1, 2, and 3 non-REM sleep; and absent during REM sleep?

    a. Serotonin.
    b. Norepinephrine.
    c. Glycine.
    d. Acetylcholine.

28. Sleep efficiency is defined as

a. the amount of time needed to go from an awake state to a sleep state.
b. the ratio of the percentage of time spent sleeping to the time spent in bed.
c. total sleep in minutes for all stages of sleep.
d. total minutes spent awake after first falling asleep and until the final awakening time.

29. A normal sinus rhythm is characterized by a P wave and QRS complex present with each beat, having a QRS interval of

a. 0.04-0.11 seconds.
b. 0.15-0.25 seconds.
c. 0.2-0.9 seconds.
d. 2-3 seconds.

30. The Berlin questionnaire (1996) asks about which of the following?

a. Daytime tiredness or fatigue: presence, frequency, and occurrences while driving (falling asleep).
b. Hypertension.
c. Snoring: presence, characteristics, frequency, impact on bed partner and others, and apneic episodes.
d. All of the above.

31. Central sleep apnea is characterized by which of the following?

a. Increased oxygen saturation.
b. Absence of chest wall and abdominal movements during apneic periods.
c. Snoring that is usually very loud.
d. All of the above.

32. Dopamine agonists, opioids, anticonvulsants, and benzodiazepines are therapeutic interventions for

a. restless legs syndrome.
b. obstructive sleep apnea.
c. insomnia.
d. circadian rhythm sleep disorder.

33. During a multiple sleep latency test, how is sleep onset defined?

a. Three or more epochs of stage N1 or a single epoch of the other sleep stages.
b. When spindles are seen.
c. The first 30-second epoch in which alpha begins to subside.
d. The first 30-second epoch in which there is more than 15 seconds of cumulative sleep.

34. Where are the reference electrodes M1 and M2 placed on the head?

a. On the earlobes.
b. On either side of the Cz electrode placement.
c. In the preauricular area behind the ear.
d. Either on the earlobes or in the preauricular area behind the ear.

35. Patients that suffer from frequent sinus infections should be advised not to wear which of the following masks?

    a. Nasal masks.
    b. Nasal-pillow masks.
    c. Full face masks.
    d. Orofacial masks.

36. What is the recommended minimum/maximum differential for IPAP and EPAP settings during a BiPAP titration?

    a. 4–6 cm apart.
    b. 6–10 cm apart.
    c. 4–10 cm apart.
    d. 2–8 cm apart.

37. The physician's orders indicate that the patient is in the lab for a CPAP titration study; however, the patient insists he has never had a sleep study before. All of the following solutions would be acceptable to resolve this situation EXCEPT

    a. call a member of the lab management team.
    b. run the study according to the physician's orders without verification.
    c. attempt to contact the ordering physician, and verify the medical intent.
    d. look through the patient's chart for evidence of a previous study.

38. An artifact that results from salt bridges is most likely caused by

    a. incorrect measuring.
    b. prepping too large an area.
    c. allowing tape or gauze from different locations to make contact.
    d. all of the above.

39. Which electrode site is found halfway between the inion and the nasion?

    a. P4
    b. Fz
    c. Cz
    d. Pz

40. What condition would require a full face mask or oral mask during a CPAP study?

    a. The patient is a mouth breather.
    b. The patient feels congested.
    c. The patient has a deviated septum.
    d. The patient is claustrophobic.

41. All of the following are indications that a patient is entering stage N1 sleep from the wake stage EXCEPT

    a. there is a reduction in chin EMG amplitude.
    b. alpha frequencies in occipital channels have reduced or stopped entirely.
    c. the eyes roll gently.
    d. the eyes mirror the EEG frequencies.

42. Where must the conductive paste be placed in relation to the gold cup wire?

    a. Inside the gold cup.
    b. Around the outside of the gold cup.
    c. Between the gold cup and gauze or tape.
    d. Inside and around the outside of the gold cup.

43. True statements about how a technician should respond when a patient experiences a seizure include all of the following EXCEPT

    a. remove any objects nearby that could injure the patient.
    b. hold the patient down to prevent injury.
    c. avoid placing anything in the patient's mouth or prying the mouth open.
    d. avoid giving liquids during or just after the seizure.

44. On which muscles are the leg EMG leads placed, and how far apart should they be from one another?

    a. Calf muscles, 4 cm apart.
    b. Anterior tibialis, 6 cm apart.
    c. Calf muscles, 2 cm apart.
    d. Anterior tibialis, 2 cm apart.

45. Which channels are necessary in the software montage for a multiple sleep latency test?

    I. Leg EMG
    II. Chin EMG
    III. EOG monitors
    IV. EEG leads
    V. EKG monitors
    VI. SpO$_2$

    a. I, II, III, and V
    b. I, III, IV, and V
    c. II, III, IV, and V
    d. II, III, IV, and VI

46. Which of the following EEG waveforms are in the correct order from the highest to the lowest frequency?

    a. Beta, delta, theta, and alpha.
    b. Delta, alpha, beta, and theta.
    c. Beta, theta, delta, and alpha.
    d. Beta, alpha, theta, and delta.

47. According to guidelines from the American Academy of Sleep Medicine, what is required to run a multiple sleep latency test?

    a. A signed form from the patient stating they slept 8 hours the night before.
    b. An overnight PSG recording.
    c. A family member who witnessed the patient sleeping the night before.
    d. Observation of the patient for 24 hours before the study.

48. When applying supplemental oxygen to a CPAP titration study, the setting at which the oxygen should be started is

 a. 1 L/min.
 b. 2 L/min.
 c. 3 L/min.
 d. 5 L/min.

49. Occurrences in a sleep study that must be scored include all of the following EXCEPT

 a. sleep stages.
 b. position changes.
 c. arousals.
 d. leg movements.

50. How frequently should the technician check on patients and be available for any requests they may have?

 a. Every 15 minutes.
 b. Every 30 minutes.
 c. Every 60 minutes.
 d. Throughout the entire study.

Questions 51–56 pertain to the following table:

Table 1. Data Collected from a Sleep Study of a 42-Year-Old Male Patient

Epoch Numbers		Number of Events	
Lights on	760	Total obstructive apneas	85
Lights out	25	Total central apneas	0
Sleep onset	52	Total mixed apneas	30
REM onset	272	Total hypopneas	45
Total wake	210	Total arousals	220
Total stage 1	35	Total periodic leg movements (PLMs)	95
Total stage 2	330	Total PLMs with arousals	60
Total stage delta	55		
Total REM stage	105		

51. Using the data in Table 1, what is the total recording time?

 a. 367.5 minutes.
 b. 380 minutes.
 c. 735 minutes.
 d. None of the above.

52. Using the data in Table 1, what is the total sleep time?

 a. 105 minutes.
 b. 210 minutes.
 c. 262.5 minutes.
 d. 525 minutes.

53. **Using the data in Table 1, what is the sleep efficiency?**

    a. 66.0%.
    b. 71.4%.
    c. 74.1%.
    d. 78.4%.

54. **Using the data in Table 1, what is the sleep latency?**

    a. 13.5 minutes.
    b. 15.0 minutes.
    c. 26.0 minutes.
    d. Not enough data are given.

55. **Using the data in Table 1, what is the percentage of stage REM sleep?**

    a. 5.0%.
    b. 12%.
    c. 20%.
    d. Impossible to calculate.

56. **Using the data in Table 1, what is the patient's apnea–hypopnea index?**

    a. 0.8/hr.
    b. 18.3/hr.
    c. 36.6/hr.
    d. 61.0/hr.

57. **At what age does the American Academy of Sleep Medicine begin considering a patient under the adult scoring guidelines?**

    a. 10 years of age.
    b. 13 years of age.
    c. 16 years of age.
    d. 18 years of age.

58. **Flow monitoring devices that may be used on patients during a sleep study include all of the following EXCEPT**

    a. a nasal/oral thermistor or thermocouple.
    b. a pressure transducer airflow.
    c. a transcutaneous carbon dioxide (CO_2) monitor.
    d. an end tidal CO_2 monitor.

59. **The artifacts that are most likely to cause high-amplitude, low-frequency waves seen on the EEG are**

    a. EKG artifacts.
    b. 60-Hz artifacts.
    c. respiratory artifacts.
    d. EOG artifacts.

60. Which of the following low-frequency/high-frequency filter settings appropriately isolate the significant frequency ranges in the EEG channels?

    a. 0.1/35.
    b. 0.3/35.
    c. 0.5/35.
    d. 1.0/35.

61. Delta waves must be how many microvolts (μV) in amplitude to count toward stage N3 sleep percentages?

    a. 75 μV.
    b. 30 μV.
    c. 100 μV.
    d. 55 μV.

62. Correct statements about acceptable PAP titration results include all of the following EXCEPT

    a. it reduces the respiratory disturbance index (RDI) to less than 5 for at least a 15-minute duration and should include supine REM sleep at the selected pressure that is not continually interrupted by spontaneous arousals or awakenings.
    b. it reduces the RDI to 10 or less or by 50% of the baseline RDI less than 15 and should include supine REM sleep that is not continually interrupted by spontaneous arousals or awakenings at the selected pressure.
    c. it reduces the RDI to less than 5 for at least a 15-minute duration without supine sleep seen at the selected pressure.
    d. it does not reduce the RDI to 10 or less but reduces the RDI by 50% from baseline in severe patients.

63. What causes EKG artifacts in the EEG and EOG channels?

    a. Improper EKG patch placement.
    b. M1 and M2 being placed directly on the auricular branch of the posterior auricular artery.
    c. Incorrect filter settings on the EEG and EOG channels.
    d. None of the above.

64. Which of the following arrhythmias qualifies as a medical emergency?

    a. Premature atrial beats.
    b. Unsustained sinus tachycardia.
    c. Junctional escape rhythm.
    d. Third-degree atrioventricular block.

65. Which of the following is a safe guideline for identifying what actions and observations should be documented by the technician?

    a. Document only things the physician cannot identify through viewing the raw data.
    b. When in doubt, document everything; the technician can never document too much.
    c. Only document actions that are listed in policy and procedures specifically.
    d. Only document things patients do that are out of the ordinary.

66. When should the technician review the patient's history and become familiar with any special needs the patient may have?

    a. Before the patient arrives.
    b. While the patient gets ready for bed.
    c. After the patient is hooked up.
    d. While the study is running.

67. The proper way to score a major body movement–dominated epoch in a recording is described by which of the following?

    a. If an alpha rhythm is present for part of the epoch, score as stage wake.
    b. If no alpha rhythm can be discerned, but an epoch of stage wake either precedes or follows the epoch with a major body movement, score as stage wake.
    c. If no alpha rhythm and no stage wake precedes or follows the epoch, score the epoch as the same stage as the epoch that follows it.
    d. All of the above statements are true about scoring major body movement epochs.

68. Reasons to alert the physician of an immediate need to review a patient's study include all of the following EXCEPT

    a. the apnea–hypopnea index is more than 80, but there is insufficient time to perform a CPAP titration.
    b. the patient has a history of hypertension, diabetes, and congestive heart failure.
    c. severe desaturations and cardiac arrhythmias are associated with the apneic events.
    d. there is a periodic leg movement index of over 40.

69. The capnograph is reading zero on the patient and on the technician who tests the cannula. The most likely cause of the equipment failure is

    a. the power is off.
    b. the patient's secretions have reached the infrared portion of the tubing.
    c. the patient is a mouth-breather.
    d. the cannula is faulty.

70. Asking the patient to look left/right and up/down during biocalibrations is intended to mimic which common situation found during healthy sleep?

    a. Eye movements in REM sleep.
    b. Seizure activity.
    c. Gently rolling eyes seen in stage N1 sleep.
    d. Bruxism.

71. During healthy respirations in NREM sleep, the brain relies on the hypoxic drive to trigger breaths. The hypoxic drive triggers a breath when which blood gas increases sufficiently?

    a. Oxygen.
    b. Carbon dioxide.
    c. Oxygen partial pressure.
    d. Bicarbonate.

72. Central sleep apnea can be seen in all of the following sleep stages EXCEPT

    a. N1.

    b. REM.

    c. N2.

    d. N3 (slow-wave sleep).

73. What can be done to improve sweat sway artifacts on the EEG and EOG channels?

    a. Increase the temperature in the room.

    b. Add extra paste to the electrodes.

    c. Decrease the temperature in the room, and turn on a fan.

    d. Reapply the affected electrodes.

74. When fitting a patient with a CPAP mask, it is important to check that

    a. the mask covers the nose and mouth adequately.

    b. air is moving through the tubing.

    c. there is no leak above clinical levels escaping from the mask.

    d. the upper lip area has space to move.

75. During observation of a PSG, which of the following positions yields more severe obstructive events and louder snoring?

    a. Supine.

    b. Prone.

    c. Right.

    d. Left.

Answer Key and Explanations for Test #1

1. B: The correct answer is excessive fragmentary myoclonus (EFM). Scoring requires that the activity continue for at least 20 minutes of non-REM sleep, with at least five EMG potentials per minute. EFM appears to be benign. The duration of an activity burst is usually 150 ms or less, but it may be greater than 150 ms if twitching is obvious. By contrast, bruxism is the grinding of the teeth. In REM sleep behavior disorder (RBD), some transient muscle activity (usually involving the muscles of the hands, feet, or mouth) often occurs during REM sleep. In addition, some large muscle activity may occur, but does not involve muscle activity across joints. Rhythmic movement disorder (RMD) is common in infants beginning at approximately six months of age and continuing until two to three years of age; it is rare after age five unless a patient has a central nervous system injury. It often includes rocking, head rolling, or head banging. Some children may also have leg banging and body rolling. Most often, RMD occurs either during stage W, when the patient is very drowsy, or during stage 1 non-REM sleep. The rhythmic movements may be accompanied by humming.

2. C: The cEMG is the chin electromyogram. By recording the muscle tone of the chin muscles, it helps the observer to identify REM sleep (during which there is a reduced muscle tone). The cEMG provides information about snoring, which causes artifacts on cEMG. In addition, it provides information on teeth grinding, which causes muscular movement. It is the EEG (not the cEMG) that provides information on the electrical activity within the brain. Through the use of scalp electrodes, the EEG measures electrical brain activity in order to rule out seizure disorders and to determine sleep-wake state characteristics.

3. C: The correct answer is that if one is not asleep within 20 minutes of going to bed, he or she should get up to do something relaxing until feeling sleepy. According to the principles of good sleep hygiene, the bed should only be used for sleeping and sex. Good sleep hygiene involves avoiding activities that interfere with sleep, such as smoking, drinking alcohol or caffeinated beverages, watching TV in bed right before trying to go to sleep, and taking naps during the day.

4. A: The hypothalamus has a role in almost all body processes, including autonomic functions, homeostasis, endocrine processes, emotions, and the regulation of sleep. By contrast, mamillary bodies are active in the memory of smells. The hippocampus is a brain region that is responsible for organizing and processing memories and spatial relationships, and for regulating emotions. The posterior pituitary gland stores and secretes oxytocin and antidiuretic hormone.

5. B: The correct answer is that morning/evening questionnaires ask the patient to indicate the five consecutive hours during the day that the patient would prefer to work. A morning/evening questionnaire asks the patient to indicate how he or she feels in the morning after going to sleep at 11 PM. In addition, it asks the patient to assess his or her appetite one-half hour after awakening.

6. D: The correct answer is 90%. One criterion for scoring pediatric obstructive sleep apnea is that there is a 90% or greater decrease in amplitude for 90% or more of events, compared to baseline.

7. A: The correct answer is generalized tonic-clonic seizures. Generalized tonic-clonic seizures may affect part of or the entire brain, causing alterations or loss of consciousness and convulsions. Interictal epileptiform activity (IEA) refers to epileptic-like changes in the EEG that commonly occur between seizures and during sleep. Primary generalized myoclonic epilepsy is characterized by brief jerking motions. Amyotrophic lateral sclerosis (ALS) is a degenerative disease of the motor neurons from the anterior horns of the spinal cord and the motor nuclei in the lower brainstem. ALS is characterized by increasing muscle weakness, spasticity, twitching, fatigue, and lack of

120

coordination. The symptoms of West syndrome include brain damage, resulting in infantile spasms, intellectual disability, and interictal EEG hypsarrhythmia.

8. D: The correct answer is 9-35. The Fatigue Severity Scale contains nine statements related to fatigue. The patient is required to score each statement on a scale of 1 to 7 (in which 1 is *strongly disagree* and 7 is *strongly agree*). Examples of the statements include: "I become fatigued easily," "I cannot adequately carry out all of my duties and responsibilities because of fatigue," and "My work, social, and family life suffer because of my fatigue." The scores for each statement are added together, with a score between 9 and 35 considered to be in the normal range. Scores above 35 suggest a high degree of fatigue.

9. C: The correct answer is that missed respirations associated with arousal, awakening, or desaturation of 3% or more are NOT part of scoring pediatric obstructive sleep apneas.. The scoring for central sleep apnea includes a duration of 20 or more seconds or a duration of two or more missed respirations (or equivalent), associated with arousal, awakening, or desaturation of 3% or more.

10. B: The correct answer is beta waves. Delta waves are slow waves (1–4 Hz), with an amplitude of more than 75 μV, and are present in stage 3 non-REM (slow-wave) sleep in adults. Delta waves occur in the waking state of newborns and young children and may occur in adults who are intoxicated or have schizophrenia or dementia. Vertex waves are commonly found negative deflections, with amplitude typically ranging from 50–150 μV. Vertex waves are most noticeable from the vertex and frontal leads. They may have sharp contours and occur in repetitive episodes (particularly in children). By contrast, theta waves have a frequency of 4–6 Hz and oscillations of varying amplitude, and are most easily seen with central and temporal leads. Theta waves frequently occur during daydreaming and self-hypnotic states, occur in stage 1 non-REM sleep, and may occur during arousals.

11. C: The correct answer is high impedance. A skin rash can change the skin's electrical signal. When this occurs, the technician should reposition the electrode, avoiding the irritated skin. By contrast, vibration may cause high-frequency artifacts. Swallowing can result in slow waves on EEG, and the blink produces slow waves on EOG. Eye muscle abnormality can cause a spike on EEG.

12. A: Pulse oximetry measures arterial oxygen saturation (SpO_2). By contrast, anterior tibialis electromyograms (atEMGs) monitor electrical activity in the leg muscles. When the leg muscles are relaxed, electrical activity is not present. With movement, electrical activity increases. The EOG records both vertical and horizontal eye movements and helps the observer to identify periods of REM sleep. Microphones or piezo sensors are used to indicate the degree and duration of snoring.

13. D: Statements A-C are all true. Periodic limb movements of sleep are scored as either events or series. It is a series (not an event) that requires four or more consecutive leg movements with the interval between movements ranging from 5-90 seconds. Leg movements that involve both legs are counted as one movement if they occur within 5 seconds of one another.

14. D: As air becomes cooler, its ability to hold water decreases. As a result, condensation begins to form in the tubing. This causes audible gurgling and decreased pressure, which are important to avoid in order for effective therapy to occur. One solution is to increase (not decrease) the room temperature by 5 to 6 degrees at night. Other potential solutions include using heated tubing and reducing the level of humidification. Another potential solution is to insulate the tubing to reduce the effects of ambient temperature.

15. B: Liquid oxygen is maintained at 21 psi, not 18 psi. It is true that it is stored at temperatures of -183°C in special cryogenic containers that oxygen evaporates as the tanks slowly warm, and that touching the fill valve can result in burns.

16. D: The correct answer is six hours or more. It is necessary to note the exact start and stop time for the polysomnogram (PSG). Insurance may not pay for an incomplete PSG, so all interruptions should be noted (e.g., an emergency that necessitates ending the study early).

17. D: The multiple sleep latency test (MSLT) includes five nap periods, not seven. The first nap period is within three hours of a nocturnal polysomnogram, and then spaced at two hours after the beginning of the preceding nap. It is true that the patient must not smoke within 30 minutes of starting a nap and that physiological calibrations are performed five minutes prior to the onset of the nap period. Also, a patient should stop using stimulants two weeks prior to the MSLT, so that the stimulants do not interfere with the results of the test.

18. B: The correct answer is that supraventricular tachycardia may be episodic, with periods of normal heart rate and rhythm between episodes. It originates in the atria, not the ventricles. The QRS complex appears normal. The P wave is present, but it may not be clearly defined since it may be obscured by the preceding T wave.

19. D: Stage 2 non-REM sleep is characterized on EEG by low-voltage (not high-voltage) activity with mixed frequency. Stage 2 is characterized by intervening periods between K complexes or sleep spindles of less than three minutes that are unrelated to arousal. Delta activity is less than 20% of the epoch. Also, normal K-complex activity is 1–3 per minute in young adults. Arousal may be indicated by abrupt K-complex clusters and delta waves.

20. C: For patients who use nasal masks (as opposed to oronasal masks), nasal pillows must fit snugly into each nostril. With oronasal masks, there is a greater chance of air leakage than with nasal masks. Oronasal masks cover both the nose and the mouth, so they are often more effective than nasal masks. However, oronasal masks are often less comfortable for the patient than nasal masks.

21. C: The correct answer is that one criterion for scoring pediatric respiratory effort-related arousals is that there is a 50% or more reduction in nasal pressure, compared to baseline. Additional scoring criteria for nasal pressure are a flattening of nasal pressure waveforms; evidence of snoring, snoring respirations, increased carbon dioxide partial pressure (pCO_2), or observable increased respiratory effort; and a duration of two or more respirations (or an equivalent duration of two respirations based upon baseline recordings).

22. C: The correct answer is 95-98% oxygen saturation. This is equal to a normal PaO_2 of 80–100 mm Hg. Levels that are lower than 40 mm Hg are dangerous.

23. A: The correct answer is that Cheyne-Strokes breathing can occur with damage to the central nervous system, hyperventilation, and heart failure. Pulse oximetry during the respirations shows a wave-like waveform as saturation begins to fall during the apneic period and then rises during periods of rapid respirations. One criterion for scoring the respirations is consecutive cycles of a crescendo-to-decrescendo breathing pattern that lasts for a minimum of ten (not two) consecutive minutes. One criterion for scoring the respirations is consecutive cycles of a crescendo-to-decrescendo breathing pattern that include five (not three) central apneas or central hypopneas per hour of sleep.

24. D: The correct answer is 13 hours. A five-year-old child requires 11 hours, and an eight-year-old child requires 10.25 hours. An eleven-year-old child requires a daily 9.5 hours of sleep.

25. D: Diet and exercise to control obesity is a therapeutic intervention for obstructive sleep apnea (OSA), but not for narcolepsy. OSA symptoms tend to lessen with weight loss. By contrast, selective serotonin reuptake inhibitors (SSRIs) and tricyclic antidepressants (TCAs) are therapeutic interventions for narcolepsy. Amphetamine-like drugs such as methylphenidate decrease sleepiness during the daytime and reduce daytime sleeping.

26. D: The correct answer is bending at the waist to reach items. Such bending should be avoided; rather, the technician should stoop down with the knees bent. It is very important for sleep technicians to use proper body mechanics, in order to prevent back injury when helping patients to change positions during the night. It is important to avoid pushing or pulling with the arms. Instead, the technician should use the entire body to relieve strain on the arms and back. Furthermore, the technician should use a step stool to reach items that are out of reach (as opposed to stretching overhead). Rather than twisting to lift, the technician should stand near the person or item to be lifted, bend his or her knees and hips, and use the muscles in his or her legs to support weight rather than using his or her back or arms to support the weight.

27. B: The correct answer is norepinephrine. In order to maintain the awake state, levels of norepinephrine increase. Levels of norepinephrine decrease during stages 1, 2, and 3 non-REM sleep. During REM sleep, norepinephrine is absent. Serotonin levels rise during the awake state but decrease during non-REM and REM sleep. This helps to regulate the onset of sleep, with the lowest levels present during REM sleep. During REM sleep, glycine levels rise to inhibit the motor nervous system at the spinal cord to cause atonia. Acetylcholine levels rise during the wake state and during REM sleep, and decrease during stages 1, 2, and 3 non-REM sleep.

28. B: *Sleep efficiency* (SE) is defined as the ratio of the percentage of time spent sleeping to the time spent in bed. *Sleep onset latency* (SOL) determines the amount of time needed to go from an awake state to a sleep state. *Total sleep time* (TST) is defined as the total sleep in minutes for all stages of sleep. *Wake-after sleep onset* (WASO) is defined as the total minutes spent awake after first falling asleep and until the final awakening time.

29. A: The correct answer is 0.04-0.11 seconds. In addition, a normal sinus rhythm is characterized by each beat having a P:QRS ratio of 1:1 and a P-R interval of 0.12–0.20 seconds.

30. D: The correct answer is *all of the above*. The Berlin questionnaire (1996) is most often used for screening people who are at risk for obstructive sleep apnea (OSA). Occasionally, it is used to assess a patient's progress after the onset of treatment with positive airway pressure. The questionnaire contains a total of fourteen questions in three categories. The questions in category 1 assess snoring (presence, characteristics, frequency, impact on bed partner and others, and apneic episodes). The questions in category 2 assess daytime tiredness or fatigue: presence, frequency, and occurrences while driving (falling asleep). The questions in category 3 assess whether hypertension is present or body mass index (BMI) is 30 kg/m² or more. A patient is classified as *high risk* or *low risk* based upon positive findings in the three different categories. A patient who is classified as high risk is one for whom positive scores are found in two or three categories. A patient who is considered low risk is one for whom positive scores are found in no more than one category.

31. B: In central sleep apnea, apneic episodes occur without obstruction of the upper airway. Central sleep apnea typically results from neurological or cardiac disorders that cause impairment of ventilation. In central sleep apnea, reduced oxygen saturation is present. There is an absence of chest wall and abdominal movements during the apneic periods. Snoring is usually mild (as opposed to obstructive sleep apnea, which is characterized by loud snoring).

32. A: The correct answer is restless legs syndrome (RLS). Dopamine agonists, opioids, and anticonvulsants may reduce symptoms of RLS. The benzodiazepine clonazepam depresses central nervous system activity; it allows the patient to sleep more but does not fully eradicate RLS.

33. D: In a multiple sleep latency test (MSLT), sleep onset is the first 30-second epoch in which there is more than 15 seconds of cumulative sleep. For the purposes of determining how long the MSLT nap will last and sleep latency, sleep onset is defined as the first epoch that has more than 50% of any stage of sleep in it. Arousals and interruptions do not negate the possibility of sleep onset as long as the 15 seconds of total sleep is reached within that 30-second epoch.

34. D: The most common placement is the preauricular location behind the ears. For patients with an abundance of fat tissue or an exceptional EEG artifact, the M1 and M2 can be attached to the earlobes instead. The integrity of the entire EEG for the study relies on the proper placement of these reference electrodes.

35. B: Nasal-pillow masks deliver the whole of the PAP pressure into the nasal passages and directly into the sinuses at the back of the nose. For patients who have easily irritated sinuses and nasal passages, the nasal-pillow design causes them a lot of discomfort. Patients should be screened for sinus issues before determining the appropriate mask selection.

36. C: During a BiPAP titration, the American Academy of Sleep Medicine (AASM) recommends that the IPAP and EPAP remain at least 4 cm apart; this is an industry standard. For special circumstances and complicated patients, the AASM recommends the spread between the IPAP and EPAP to go no higher than 10 cm apart. It is important to understand that any differential above 6 cm apart will more closely resemble manual ventilation of the patient's breathing as opposed to 4–6 cm apart, which is standard BiPAP. Greater than 6 cm apart is a less common differential typically used to assist patients in breathing excess carbon dioxide or special treatment of complex sleep apnea. These complex titrations should not be done without guidance and proper training.

37. B: A study should never begin without order verification when discrepancies are suspected. It is important to avoid telling patients that they are confused or mistaken about their own medical history, even if it is true. The correct course of action is to call management about the discrepancy, and follow up with the physician in case verbal alterations to the orders are required.

38. D: Incorrect measurement can cause leads to be too close together, and prepping a site that is larger than the electrode may allow the prep solution to connect multiple electrodes. Allowing tape or gauze to overlap can also connect multiple electrodes. If an artifact is severe, the stage of sleep will be difficult or impossible to discern.

39. C: P4 is not on the inion/nasion line at all. Fz is 30% up from the nasion, and Pz is 30% up from the inion. Cz is the electrode found 50% up from both the inion and the nasion at the top of the head. Odd locations, such as F3, are located on the left side of the head, and the even-numbered corresponding positions, such as F4, are on the right side of the head.

40. C: Most patients suffering from sleep apnea breathe through their mouth periodically during the night in an attempt to catch up on deprived oxygen. Healthy patients who are able to inhale through their nose while awake should be able to inhale through their nose while asleep when obstructive events are eliminated with CPAP machines. Congestion is a temporary inconvenience quickly remedied with sprays or the humidity setting on the CPAP machine, not full face masks. Most patients who are claustrophobic or anxious are going to prefer the smallest and least invasive mask. A deviated septum, however, is a medical condition in which the sinuses and bone have shifted to block the passage of air either partially or entirely through the nasal passages; in this case, a full face mask or oral mask would be necessary.

41. D: Muscle activity decreases in the chin channel when patients enter N1 sleep from stage wake. Alpha is only present in wake when the eyes are closed, so as a patient falls asleep the alpha frequency is no longer present in the occipital channels. Gently rolling eyes are an indicator of stage N1, while eyes mirroring the EEG are an indication of stage N2 or N3.

42. A: While the paste can be in other areas to aid in keeping the wire in place, the paste must be inside the gold cup wire. The paste is conductive, and the connection it makes with the skin is conducted through the paste and directly into the gold cup wire.

43. B: Never attempt to touch, hold, or restrain a patient suffering from a seizure. The technician should remove any objects around the patient that may cause injury because of the uncontrollable movements of the seizure. The technician may place pillows or other padding in areas where there is a possibility of injury.

44. D: Leads intended to monitor muscle activity in the legs are placed on the anterior tibialis muscle in line with one another with 2-cm spacing between the two leads placed on each leg. The anterior tibialis is the first muscle group when starting on the shin bone, just below the knee, and sliding fingers outward not inward.

45. C: According to the guidelines of the American Academy of Sleep Medicine entitled "Practice Parameters for Clinical Use of the Multiple Sleep Latency Test" and "The Maintenance of Wakefulness Test," "The conventional recording montage for the multiple sleep latency test (MSLT) includes central EEG (C3–A2, C4–A1) and occipital (O1–A2, O2–A1) derivations, left and right eye EOGs, mental/submental EMGs, and an EKG." The technician monitors sleep onset and REM onset during a MSLT study; for this reason, the EEG and chin EMG are crucial. Muscle activity in the legs and oxygen saturation are extraneous and inconsequential to the MSLT results.

46. D: Frequencies of waveforms are: beta, more than 13 Hz; alpha, 8–13 Hz; theta, 3.5–7.5 Hz; and delta, 3 Hz or less. Answer D has the four waveforms listed in order from highest frequency to lowest frequency. A commonly accepted acronym, DTABS, helps test takers remember the order of frequencies from lowest to highest: delta, theta, alpha, beta, and spindles.

47. B: While a physician can skip this step, to be in line with "Practice Parameters for Clinical Use of the Multiple Sleep Latency Test (MSLT)" and the "Maintenance of Wakefulness Test," physicians need to adhere to the following requirement: "The MSLT must be performed immediately following a PSG recorded during the individual's major sleep period. The use of MSLT to support a diagnosis of narcolepsy is suspect if total sleep time on the night before the sleep study is less than 6 hours. The test should not be performed after a split-night sleep study (combination of diagnostic and therapeutic studies in a single night)."

48. A: The guidelines of the American Academy of Sleep Medicine for the application of supplemental oxygen and PAP titration state that all qualifying conditions for the application of oxygen should be started with only 1 L/min. The supplemental oxygen can only be increased in 1 L increments from then on until a consistent range of 88%–94% SpO_2 is achieved.

49. B: Although it is a good practice to document in the study when the patient changes position, it cannot be scored within the four core parameters required by the scoring guidelines of the American Academy of Sleep Medicine. These four parameters are: sleep stages, arousals, respiratory events, and periodic leg movements.

50. D: The technician is responsible for monitoring patients' physiological data throughout the entire study. While monitoring the data, the technician should be in full contact with patients both audibly and visually in the event that they need assistance.

51. A: Recording time within a PSG is the time from "lights out" to "lights on"; all other recording data are superfluous to the study. The formula for finding total sleep time is as follows:

(Lights on epoch # – Lights out epoch #)/2

In this data set that would be:

(760 – 25)/2 = 367.5

During report generation, all times are converted into minutes. The total epochs of recording time are divided by 2 to get the minutes. Each epoch is 30 seconds long, so two epochs are equal to 1 minute.

52. C: Total sleep time (TST) is the total number of minutes the patient spends asleep between "lights out" and lights on. The formula for TST is:

(Total all sleep epochs)/2

In this data set this would be:

(35 + 330 + 55 + 105)/2 = 262.5 minutes

Paying attention to the requested answer measurement is important, while the answer is 525 epochs, it is not 525 minutes because an epoch is only 30 seconds long.

53. B: Sleep efficiency is the percentage of the recording time in which the patient is asleep. The formula for sleep efficiency is:

[Total sleep time (TST)/total recording time (TRT)] x 100

In the previous two questions the TST and TRT were calculated. For sleep efficiency, the percentage is the requested answer measurement. As a rule of thumb, when finding a percentage, it is necessary to multiply by 100 after dividing two numbers. In this case, it is as follows:

(262.5/367.5) x 100 = 71.4%

54. A: Sleep latency is defined as the time it takes for a patient to fall asleep. Sleep onset data are given in the table for the purpose of this calculation. As with all the other calculations, the data prior to "lights out" are extraneous and not used. So sleep latency is the time from "lights out" until sleep onset. The formula for this calculation is as follows:

(Sleep onset – lights out)/2

In this example that is:

$$(52 - 25)/2 = 13.5 \text{ minutes}$$

55. C: The percentage of REM sleep in comparison to all other sleep stages is the result that a report generator would give. The formula for finding the percentage of any stage is the same only changing the number for the specific total time for that sleep stage. The formula is as follows:

[Total stage REM/total sleep time (TST)] x 100

For this example, a REM percentage is needed, but any total stage time divided by TST x 100 will yield that stage's percentage. In this case, it is as follows:

$$(52.5/262.5) \times 100\% = 20\%$$

When a percentage is the requested result, multiplying by 100 is necessary.

56. C: The apnea–hypopnea index (AHI) is a calculation of the number of total apneic and hypopneic events that occur per hour. The formula for AHI is as follows:

[Total apneas and hypopneas/total sleep time (TST)] x 60

This is why TST is calculated in minutes; if TST is used in epochs or any other measure of time, the formula will not work. For this example, this means the following:

$$(160/262.5) \times 60 = 36.6/\text{hr}$$

If time is requested for the answer, it is in minutes, and the formula is divided by 2; if the question asks for a percentage, the formula is multiplied by 100; and if it is an index, it is per hour and multiplied by 60.

57. B: According to the guidelines of the American Academy of Sleep Medicine, the criteria written and outlined for children is specifically for patients under the age of 13. This age was chosen to separate pediatric patients from adult patients because it is the average age of the onset of puberty.

58. C: All of the answers except for a transcutaneous carbon dioxide (CO_2) monitor are devices placed in the nose to monitor various attributes of the patient's breathing. A thermistor measures temperatures of breaths; a pressure transducer airflow measures the volume of breaths; and an end tidal measures retention of CO_2. Transcutaneous CO_2 is not measured often during a PSG because of its inherent discomfort: it is measured through the skin and is not derived from the patient's breath.

59. C: The EKG artifacts manifest as QRS spikes in the EEG. A 60-Hz artifact is an electrical artifact at a very high frequency. An EOG artifact is not a real artifact. Respiratory artifacts sway gently in line with the flow channels, causing what looks like high-amplitude, low-frequency delta waves.

60. B: Any low-frequency filter (LFF) below 0.3 may artificially increase the amount of slow-wave sleep seen by allowing low-frequency artifacts into the study. A LFF above 0.3 will attenuate and make it impossible to see slow-wave delta sleep, which has high-frequency activity.

61. A: Delta frequency is 0.5–2 cps; it must be greater than or equal to 75 microvolts to be counted towards the 20% delta activity required to count an epoch of sleep as stage N3. Most PSG software is equipped with a device known as a voltmeter to verify the amplitude of the delta frequencies.

62. D: All answers except for D are acceptable results of a PAP titration, according to "Clinical Guidelines for the Manual Titration of Positive Airway Pressure in Patients with Obstructive Sleep

127

Apnea" from the American Academy of Sleep Medicine (AASM). The incorrect option listed involves insufficient reduction in the respiratory disturbance index (RDI) for severe patients. When a patient with severe obstructive sleep apnea is titrated, the AASM expects at least a 75% reduction of the RDI to consider it a successful titration.

63. B: M1 and M2 are placed behind the ear most of the time; they can also be placed on the ear lobe. When an EKG artifact appears in the EOG and EEG channels, it is because the technician placed the M1 and or M2 lead too far back from the ear and the reference leads are receiving data from the auricular artery. If M1 and M2 are placed appropriately, no EKG data will bleed into the EEG and EOG channels.

64. D: Third-degree atrioventricular (AV) block is the fourth most dangerous of the AV-block cardiac rhythms. Third-degree means a complete heart block. The P and the QRS waves become completely disassociated from one another. A technician witnessing this should enact their emergency policies and procedures immediately.

65. B: The technician can never document too many observations and data about the patient's sleep, actions, habits, or behaviors during the sleep study. The more information physicians have the better equipped they are to interpret the study and identify appropriate treatment options for the patient. The technician 's core task is to provide the physician with all the data and facts necessary to do this.

66. A: The technician should become familiar with any physical or mental limitations the patient may have before the first time they interact with the patient. The patient could be hurt or even needlessly aggravated if the technician is ignorant of any special needs.

67. D: With an alpha rhythm inside the major body movement epochs, the required amount to score as stage wake is less than 15 seconds, unlike normal scoring rules. Any alpha rhythm at all is sufficient to score it as stage wake. In the absence of an alpha rhythm, the major body movement is wake if any epoch before or after is wake. It is a process of elimination with the last choice being to score it as the stage of sleep that follows it.

68. D: Physicians and scoring technicians are informed of an immediate need to review a study when the patient is in dire need of therapy intervention. High apnea–hypopnea indices, severe blood oxygen drops, cardiac arrhythmias, or life-threatening comorbidities threaten the patient's health each time they sleep without PAP therapy. Periodic leg movements disrupt sleep and cause discomfort, but they are not a life-threatening sleep disorder and do not warrant a call for immediate review of the data by the physician.

69. B: Sidestream capnography monitors which measures of the carbon dioxide (CO_2) inside the device are susceptible to the infrared portion being contaminated by patient secretions or a build up of moisture and condensation. The water traps and tubing on these devices require troubleshooting and maintenance often and should be the first thing checked when faced with incorrect CO_2 values.

70. A: During biocalibration, the patient is asked to look left, then right and up then down multiple times. If the EOG placement is correct, these movements should show the same sharp, phasic eye movements found in healthy, nontonic REM sleep. Neither seizure activity nor bruxism is related to the eyes or how they move.

71. B: The hypoxic drive functions by sensing when the carbon dioxide levels in the body have peaked and a new influx of oxygen is required. This occurs only during NREM sleep. During REM sleep an entirely less precise method of erratic breathing can be seen in most patients.

72. B: Central sleep apnea is a result of the neurological respiratory control center being imbalanced or slow to respond. Central sleep apneas are cessations in breath with no effort because the brain has not yet sensed an abundance of carbon dioxide, which should trigger the body to inhale. During REM sleep this respiratory drive is ignored, and breathing continues at varying rates regardless of the brain's ability to detect blood gases accurately and promptly. This is why true central sleep apnea cannot be seen during REM sleep.

73. C: A sweat sway artifact is a large popping in the EEG and EOG channels, which is caused when patients sweat profusely. Some patients sweat no matter how cool the room is kept, and these patients are candidates for the application of antiperspirant products. If the technician can cool the room and the patient, the artifact should subside. Sweat sway can look similar to respiratory sway except it will not be in tandem with the patient's respirations.

74. C: Not every patient requires the use of a full face mask; therefore, covering the nose and mouth is not important for most masks. The air moving through the tubing is a troubleshooting issue and not directly related to how the mask fits on the patient. All other forms of comfort for the mask are secondary to the importance of leaks. If the leak is too high, then the mask is ineffective.

75. A: Optimal pressures found during CPAP titrations include the patient being supine during REM sleep for this reason. When patients turn supine, gravity works against the airway. The tongue, tissue, uvula, and jaw can fall back and cause more blockages in the upper airway. Some labs require patients to remain in the supine position for the bulk of the study, but that is not a required guideline of the American Academy of Sleep Medicine.

CPSGT Practice Test #2

1. The goals of PAP therapy include all of the following EXCEPT to

    a. improve diminished lung capacity.

    b. eliminate flow limitations in the upper airway.

    c. eliminate excessive daytime somnolence.

    d. eliminate snoring.

2. To ensure REM sleep has a chance to occur during a multiple sleep latency test nap, how long should that nap continue?

    a. 25 minutes following "lights out."

    b. 15 minutes following sleep onset.

    c. 15 minutes following "lights out."

    d. 20 minutes following sleep onset.

3. Staging choices for infants include which of the following combinations?

    a. Active REM sleep and quiet sleep.

    b. Indeterminate sleep, wake, and quiet sleep.

    c. Active REM sleep and delta sleep.

    d. Indeterminate sleep, active REM sleep, and quiet sleep.

4. Heated humidity can possibly remedy which of the following conditions seen in some patients?

    a. Patient complains of being cold.

    b. Patient mouth-breathes because of nasal congestion.

    c. Patient complains of dry throat or nose.

    d. Both B and C.

5. What is the standard length of time of each epoch during the scoring of stages in a PSG?

    a. 30 seconds.

    b. 45 seconds.

    c. 3 minutes.

    d. 10 minutes.

6. An alternating EEG pattern seen during quiet sleep in a newborn infant, consisting of both high- and low-voltage activity is termed

    a. active sleep.

    b. trace alternant.

    c. sawtooth waves.

    d. slow-wave sleep.

7. Electrical safety requires all of the following actions from a technician EXCEPT

    a. checking the conditions of wires to assure none are frayed or damaged.

    b. the application of a ground placed with the pulse oximetry probe.

    c. the application of a ground lead wire placed on the head for the PSG.

    d. keeping liquid away from all electrical components.

8. What physiological effects does CPAP have on the body?

    a. Splints the airway to allow breaths to pass through without occlusion.

    b. Improves pulmonary function.

    c. Increases blood–gas exchange efficacy.

    d. Controls respiratory rate.

9. Before a technician begins cardiopulmonary resuscitation on a patient, basic life support procedures require the technician to do which of the following?

    a. Contact a nurse for assistance.

    b. Verify the patient's unresponsiveness.

    c. Check the patient's pulse.

    d. Listen for the patient's breath.

10. Which of the following is an adequate chemical disinfectant used to clean surfaces?

    a. Oxirane.

    b. Formaldehyde.

    c. Sodium hypochlorite.

    d. Isoflurane.

11. What should the technician do if the patient awakens and complains that the pressure is too high?

    a. Switch to the pressures of BiPAP titration.

    b. Ask the patient to continue trying to return to sleep, and make no changes to the pressure.

    c. Restart pressure with one that the patient subjectively feels comfortable.

    d. Reduce pressure to no less than where obstructive apnea was eliminated.

12. Which of the following EEG frequencies can be seen during an arousal from sleep?

    a. Alpha.

    b. Theta.

    c. Any frequency over 16, excluding sleep spindles.

    d. All of the above.

13. What percentage drop in the SpO_2 data must be seen to score an obstructive event?

    a. 3% or more.

    b. 4% or more.

    c. 5% or more.

    d. No required drop in the SpO_2 channel.

14. What is the minimum time required before increasing the PAP pressure during a titration study?

    a. 5 minutes.

    b. 10 minutes.

    c. 15 minutes.

    d. 20 minutes.

15. A mixed apnea is characterized by which of the following?

a. A combination of hypopnea and obstructive characteristics.
b. A lack of respiratory effort at the start of the event where respiratory effort returns before the event ends.
c. Respiratory effort present at the start of the event where the effort ceases in the second half of the event.
d. Intermittent respiratory effort throughout an obstructive event.

16. What is the most important aspect of fielding a patient's questions in the morning following the sleep study?

a. To be positive and avoid alarming the patient.
b. To give the patient as many details about their results as possible.
c. To be vague and avoid giving any straight answers.
d. To defer all questions the patient has to the physician.

17. All of the following statements are true about the changes seen from stage N2 to N3 EXCEPT

a. sleep spindles may persist into stage N3 sleep.
b. eye movements are not typically seen.
c. EMG chin activity is often higher than in stage N2.
d. delta activity reaches 20% or more in the epoch.

18. Which of the following statements about the removal of paste residue from the patient in the morning is true?

a. The paste never needs to be removed.
b. Only remove the paste if the patient asks.
c. Remove the paste if the patient is physically unable.
d. Always remove remnants of paste from the patient's body.

19. Criteria necessary to score an arousal in NREM sleep include all of the following EXCEPT

a. a concurrent increase in chin EMG.
b. 10 seconds of sleep prior to the arousal.
c. the arousal must last at least 3 seconds.
d. frequencies greater than 16 Hz, which are not spindles, must occur.

20. Which sensors need to be cleaned and disinfected?

a. Any sensors that come into contact with the patient's bodily fluids.
b. Only sensors in the patient's nose.
c. Any sensors that come in direct contact with the patient in any location.
d. Only sensors placed in abraded locations.

21. All of the following events are required to score a leg movement EXCEPT

a. it must have a minimum duration of 0.5 seconds and a maximum duration of 10 seconds.
b. there must be an 8-microvolt (μV) increase in the EMG from baseline.
c. the end of the event is marked when the EMG remains below 2 μV up from baseline.
d. the event must be within 1 second of an ending respiratory event.

22. According to scoring guidelines of the American Academy of Sleep Medicine, which piece of equipment is used to identify hypopnea?

　　a.　Thermal sensor.
　　b.　Nasal air pressure transducer.
　　c.　Capnograph.
　　d.　None of the above.

23. What is the maximum recommended CPAP for patients under the age of 12 years?

　　a.　10 cm.
　　b.　15 cm.
　　c.　20 cm.
　　d.　25 cm.

24. Excessive transient muscle activity found in REM sleep indicates which of the following sleep disorders?

　　a.　Rhythmic movement disorder.
　　b.　Amyotrophic lateral sclerosis.
　　c.　REM behavior disorder.
　　d.　Obstructive sleep apnea disorder.

25. Which of the following does the American Academy of Sleep Medicine recommend all patients should receive before a titration begins?

　　a.　Informational packet and calming therapy.
　　b.　A course on how to use CPAP and a hands-on demonstration.
　　c.　Adequate PAP education, hands-on demonstration, careful mask fitting, and acclimatization.
　　d.　Careful mask fitting and calming therapy.

26. Required criteria for scoring an apneic event for an adult include all of the following EXCEPT

　　a.　the event lasts no longer than 30 seconds.
　　b.　there is a 90% or more drop from baseline in the thermal sensor channel.
　　c.　the duration of the event lasts at least 10 seconds.
　　d.　at least 90% of the event must meet the 90% drop from baseline criteria.

27. Where is the tape measure placed when measuring the circumference of the head?

　　a.　At all 10% up-markings on the head starting and ending at FPz.
　　b.　At the inion and nasion.
　　c.　Where the tape measure naturally lies with the patient's head shape.
　　d.　Right above the ears.

28. If the CPAP pressure is set and left below a patient's optimal pressure, what may occur?

　　a.　A decrease in patient arousals.
　　b.　REM rebound.
　　c.　Ongoing hypoventilation or hypoxemia.
　　d.　Increased compliance.

29. Which of the following is true about CPAP mask leaks?
   a.   There cannot be any clinical leak for a successful titration.
   b.   There may be some leak present, depending on the mask style.
   c.   The acceptable leak value varies from patient to patient.
   d.   Leaks should be within the manufacturer's recommended range and not causing sleep fragmentation.

30. What is the most common side effect of proper CPAP use?
   a.   Eye dryness and pain.
   b.   Dizziness.
   c.   Nasal congestion.
   d.   Tinnitus.

31. After 3 years of CPAP use, a patient returns to the sleep lab complaining of excessive daytime sleepiness. Which of the following is a possible cause for the CPAP no longer providing the patient with optimal sleep?
   a.   Excessive alcohol use.
   b.   Patient no longer has sleep apnea.
   c.   Damaged equipment.
   d.   Both A and C.

32. Which filter would be used to adjust the rise time of a signal?
   a.   The LFF.
   b.   The HFF.
   c.   The gain.
   d.   The sensitivity.

33. Where is the O1 lead located in relation to the T3 lead?
   a.   Left and behind, 25% of the total circumference of the head.
   b.   Right and behind, 25% of the total circumference of the head.
   c.   Left and behind, 20% of the total circumference of the head.
   d.   Right and behind, 20% of the total circumference of the head.

34. _____ is measured in Hertz (Hz) and _____ in microvolts (uV).
   a.   Amplitude, frequency
   b.   Amplitude, sensitivity
   c.   Frequency, sensitivity
   d.   Frequency, amplitude

35. In polysomnography, sensitivity is generally measured in
   a.   uV/mm.
   b.   uV/cm.
   c.   uV/in.
   d.   Hz/mm.

36. What is the most likely sensitivity setting for the EEG in a polysomnogram?

- a. 3 uV/mm.
- b. 15 uV/mm.
- c. 7 uV/mm.
- d. 1 uV/mm.

37. Periodic limb movements in sleep (PLMS) are defined as

- a. at least 2 movements, between 5 and 90 seconds apart, and between 0.5 and 5 seconds in duration for each movement.
- b. at least 4 movements, between 5 and 90 seconds apart, and between 1 and 10 seconds in duration for each movement.
- c. at least 4 movements, between 5 and 90 seconds apart, and between 0.5 and 10 seconds in duration for each movement.
- d. at least 4 movements, between 10 and 90 seconds apart, and between 0.5 and 5 seconds in duration for each movement.

38. Sleep spindles are

- a. associated with stage 3 sleep.
- b. 12–14 Hz.
- c. have specific amplitude requirements.
- d. associated with stage 1 sleep.

Use the following information to answer questions 39–44:

Lights off: 23:30
Lights on: 05:30
Sleep onset: 00:30
Total NREM sleep time (min): 230
Total REM sleep time (min): 45

39. What is the total recording time (TRT), in minutes?

- a. 275.
- b. 360.
- c. 300.
- d. 230.

40. What is the total sleep time (TST), in minutes?

- a. 275.
- b. 360.
- c. 300.
- d. 230.

41. What is the total wake time (TWT), in minutes?

- a. 25.
- b. 15.
- c. 100.
- d. 85.

42. What is the sleep efficiency (rounded to the nearest percentage)?

    a. 70%.
    b. 89%.
    c. 76%.
    d. 74%.

43. What is the percentage of REM sleep (rounded to the nearest percentage)?

    a. 20%.
    b. 16%.
    c. 15%.
    d. 84%.

44. What is the percentage of NREM sleep (rounded to the nearest percentage)?

    a. 20%.
    b. 16%.
    c. 15%.
    d. 84%.

Use the following information to answer questions 45–47:

    Sleep latencies during an MSLT:
    Nap #1: 5 minutes
    Nap #2: 4 minutes
    Nap #3: 3 minutes
    Nap #4: 4 minutes
    Nap #5: 9 minutes

45. What is the mean sleep latency for this MSLT?

    a. 5 minutes.
    b. 4 minutes.
    c. 9 minutes.
    d. 25 minutes.

46. What is the mode sleep latency of this MSLT?

    a. 5 minutes.
    b. 4 minutes.
    c. 3 minutes.
    d. 9 minutes.

47. What is the median sleep latency?

    a. 5 minutes.
    b. 4 minutes.
    c. 14.5 minutes.
    d. 4.5 minutes.

48. In which study does a patient try to stay awake in a darkened room?

    a. MSLT.
    b. MWT.
    c. NPSG.
    d. REM behavior disorder study.

49. What is hypnagogic jerk?

a. A muscle spasm during the transition from stage 1 to stage 2 sleep.
b. A muscle spasm during the transition from stage 2 to REM sleep.
c. A muscle spasm during the transition from sleep to wakefulness.
d. A muscle spasm during the transition from wakefulness to sleep.

50. A patient is snoring on CPAP at 11 cwp. What is the best course of action for the technician to take?

a. Lower the CPAP to 10 cwp.
b. Switch to BiPAP 15/10 cwp.
c. Raise the CPAP to 12 cwp.
d. Do nothing. Snoring is not treated by CPAP.

51. A patient who had no central apneas during her initial polysomnogram begins presenting with central apneas at 15 cwp on CPAP. What is the most likely cause?

a. The CPAP pressure is too low.
b. The CPAP pressure is too high.
c. There is a mask leak.
d. This is natural and isn't a concern.

52. BiPAP S/T stands for

a. bilevel positive airway pressure spontaneous/timed.
b. bilevel positive air pressure spontaneous/timed.
c. bilevel positive airway pressure synchronized/timed.
d. bilevel positive air pressure synchronized/timed.

53. Muscle artifact can be corrected by

a. decreasing the HFF.
b. decreasing the LFF.
c. moving the electrode that the artifact is appearing on.
d. either decreasing the HFF or moving the electrode that the artifact is appearing on.

54. Sweat artifact looks like

a. slow-wave sleep.
b. a solid, fuzzy bar in the electrode channel.
c. a random, sudden "popping" in the electrode channel.
d. an arousal.

55. The best way to eliminate artifact is by

a. adjusting the filters.
b. going to the problem source and replacing and reapplying the affected leads.
c. doing nothing, as they tend to resolve on their own.
d. stopping the study and reapplying all the leads.

56. K-complexes are often seen

a. in stage 1 sleep.
b. in stage 2 sleep.
c. in stage 3 sleep.
d. in REM.

57. Cataplexy is

    a. a sudden jolt or spasm when transitioning from wake to stage 1.

    b. the loss of muscle tone in REM.

    c. the loss of muscle tone that accompanies a strong emotion.

    d. a waxing or waning in respiratory flow and rate.

58. All are potential causes of central sleep apnea EXCEPT

    a. congestive heart failure.

    b. brain stem injury.

    c. obesity.

    d. neurological disease.

59. People with obstructive sleep apnea have a higher risk of

    a. stroke.

    b. COPD.

    c. hypotension.

    d. depression.

60. For Americans the most common sleep disorder is

    a. insomnia.

    b. obstructive sleep apnea.

    c. central sleep apnea.

    d. narcolepsy.

61. A 43-year-old male who is 5'8" tall and weighs 275 pounds, with no history of smoking or alcohol abuse, complains of trouble falling asleep, headaches, and daytime fatigue. His wife complains that his legs are kicking her while she is asleep. He most likely has

    a. obstructive sleep apnea.

    b. central sleep apnea.

    c. Cheyne-Stokes breathing pattern.

    d. PLMS.

62. During a CPAP titration study a patient at a CPAP pressure of 15 cm who is still snoring and having hypopneas complains that the pressure feels too high and she cannot sleep. What should the technician do?

    a. Leave the CPAP at 15 cm and wait for the patient to fall back to sleep.

    b. Lower the CPAP pressure to 13 cm and wait for the patient to fall back to sleep before raising it again.

    c. Raise the CPAP pressure to 17 cm.

    d. Switch to BiPAP of 15/11 cm and continue the titration.

63. Key things to look for in REM behavior disorder montage are

    a. muscle movements, increased chin EMG activity, and obstructive apneas in REM.

    b. muscle movements, increased chin EMG activity, and central apneas in REM.

    c. muscle movements, decreased chin EMG activity, and obstructive apneas in REM.

    d. muscle movements and increased chin EMG activity in REM.

64. REM behavior disorder is usually treated with

    a. CPAP.

    b. medications such as benzodiazepines, Sinemet, and clonidine.

    c. medications such as Ambien, Lunesta, or Sonata.

    d. medications such as Provigil, Ritalin, or Dexedrine.

65. Which of the following medications is used to treat narcolepsy?

    a. Ambien.

    b. Mirapex.

    c. Dextroamphetamine.

    d. Aspirin.

66. The technician's duties include all of the following EXCEPT

    a. providing a safe environment for the patient.

    b. giving an interpretation of the study to the patient.

    c. making sure the study is accurate.

    d. changing CPAP pressure.

67. The technician should log which patient information into the computer before the study?

    a. Medical history.

    b. Time of last nicotine intake.

    c. Study identification number.

    d. Time of arrival.

68. Antidepressants suppress which stage of sleep?

    a. Stage 1.

    b. Stage 2.

    c. Stage 3.

    d. REM.

69. Alcohol can suppress which stage(s) of sleep?

    a. Stage 2.

    b. Stage 3.

    c. NREM.

    d. Stage 1.

70. Nicotine may cause

    a. insomnia.

    b. sleep apnea.

    c. REM behavior disorder.

    d. daytime sleepiness.

71. In an EKG the P wave represents

    a. atrial depolarization.

    b. atrial contraction.

    c. ventricular depolarization.

    d. ventricular contraction.

72. In an EKG the QRS complex represents

    a. atrial contraction.
    b. ventricular repolarization.
    c. ventricular contraction.
    d. atrial depolarization.

73. In an ECG the T wave represents

    a. ventricular contraction.
    b. ventricular repolarization.
    c. atrial repolarization.
    d. atrial contraction.

74. G1 and G2 represent

    a. the first signal input and the ground lead, respectively.
    b. the ground lead and the first signal input, respectively.
    c. the first signal input and the second signal input, respectively.
    d. the ground lead and the exploring electrode, respectively.

75. What is the minimum AHI to be diagnosed with OSA?

    a. >5/hr.
    b. >3/hr.
    c. >10/hr.
    d. >15/hr.

Answer Key and Explanations for Test #2

1. A: The CPAP and BiPAP used in the sleep lab are non-invasive respiratory therapies that do not have effects on patient's lung capacity or tidal volumes. The focus of the PAP devices is to maintain the structural integrity of the airway, especially the upper airway, to prevent collapses that result in obstructive apneas and snoring.

2. B: According to the guidelines of the American Academy of Sleep Medicine for the operation of a multiple sleep latency test (MSLT), a MSLT nap continues for 15 minutes following sleep onset. The first thing for which the MSLT is looking is to see if the patient is capable of falling asleep in a 20-minute space of time. If a patient does not fall asleep within 20 minutes, the nap is ended. If the patient falls asleep during the 20-minute window, the nap continues for 15 more minutes from that time to see if REM can be reached shortly after sleep onset.

3. D: When scoring infant sleep studies, the only available options for sleep stage scoring are indeterminate sleep, active REM sleep, and quiet sleep. At around 6 months of age, pediatric scoring rules become more applicable as waveforms, such as sleep spindles, become manifested. An infant's EEG is so unlike the pediatric and adult waveforms that identifying the standard sleep stages would be impossible.

4. D: Heated humidity can be used when patients specifically complain about the drying effect of the pressure being applied to their nose and or mouth. Other times while the patient is asleep, nasal congestion may lead to problematic oral venting. In the cases of oral venting interrupting a successful titration, heated humidity can break up nasal congestion.

5. A: According to guidelines of the American Academy of Sleep Medicine entitled, "The Visual Scoring of Sleep in Adults," scoring by 30-second epochs was retained from the Rechtshaffen and Kales process of scoring sleep studies. The reason for the either 20- or 30-second view of the EEG is the ability to see the vertex spike waves, complexes, and spindles clearly enough to confirm sleep staging.

6. B: Trace alternant is the NREM sleep for infants that diminishes and becomes nonexistent between 3–6 weeks of age in healthy infants. This pattern is found in an infant's slow-wave sleep and after the first month of life; it is gradually replaced with sleep spindles.

7. B: Pulse oximetry devices are very low-voltage, passive electrical devices that do not require a ground to avoid patient electrocution. Pulse oximetry is a direct current electrical device. Frayed and exposed wires, improperly grounded surface electrodes, as well as wet equipment can electrocute a patient.

8. A: The CPAP will not increase pulmonary function in patients, and it will not improve the rate at which oxygen is transferred into the heart. However, CPAP supports the structural integrity of the airway when patients fail to hold the airway open with their own muscles. By preventing a collapse of the airway, an apneic patient will never have to struggle to reopen their airway while asleep.

9. B: According to "Basic Life Support Procedures" from the American Heart Association, health care providers should not initiate cardiopulmonary resuscitation (CPR) on conscious and responsive patients. That is not to say that a patient must be unresponsive for it to be an emergency situation; however, CPR does require the patient to be unconscious.

10. C: Oxirane is a cyclic ether used in high-level sterilization; it is not recommended for casual surface cleaning and is far too powerful for such a task. Formaldehyde is also a very powerful disinfectant and sterilant, which should only be used on critically contaminated surfaces. Isoflurane is an inhaled ether gas used in anesthetics and would not be appropriate for any surface cleaning. Sodium hypochlorite, or bleach, is a safe and appropriate chemical for surface cleaning when used according to directions.

11. C: Often patients will awaken from sleep confused and panicked at this strange new device that they forgot was on their face. The reactions commonly seen are anxiety and fear. The most important goal when facing patients who complain of the pressure being too high is for them to return to sleep. If patients cannot return to sleep, then the titration cannot continue. The technician should do whatever the patients want to instill calm and allow them to return to sleep as far as the PAP pressure is concerned, even if it does not make sense.

12. D: The guidelines of the American Academy of Sleep Medicine for scoring arousals suggest scoring them during any stage of sleep, if there is an abrupt shift of EEG frequency, including alpha, theta, or frequencies over 16 Hz (not including spindles) that last at least 3 seconds, with at least 10 seconds of stable sleep preceding the change. Arousals may be scored within epochs that are predominantly stage wake as long as there are 10 seconds of sleep before the arousal is present.

13. D: Scoring obstructive apneas only relies on the 90% for 90% of the event with respiratory effort throughout criteria. Unlike hypopneas, apneas do not require an associated drop in blood oxygen saturation to be scored. Obstructive apneas will often have desaturations associated with them, and the validity of the event should be questioned if there is not a change in the SpO_2.

14. A: According to the American Academy of Sleep Medicine, CPAP should be increased by at least 1 cm with an interval no shorter than 5 minutes. Increases in PAP do not have an immediate effect on splinting the patient's airway, so time is necessary to observe how effective the increase really was. Aside from the necessity to verify efficacy of PAP increases, if a technician raises the pressure too quickly the patient may respond with complex sleep apnea. Complex sleep apnea is a result of the patient's body rejecting the PAP pressure and refusing to initiate breaths.

15. B: A mixed apnea is a respiratory event that begins with the qualities of a central sleep apneic event. As long as any respiratory effort begins before normal breath and recovery happens, it is scored as a mixed apnea. It cannot be the opposite, and a mixed apnea in no way indicates a combination of any other respiratory events besides the above description.

16. A: While the technician should avoid giving results and diagnoses to the patient in the morning, there are certain things the technician can and should share with the patient. The only real universal guideline is to avoid using phrases that may alarm or terrify the patient. Even though technicians understand what it means to "stop breathing" during apneic events, a patient may hear those words and become terrified to sleep. Considering it may be weeks before they are treated with CPAP therapy, it would be very inconvenient for them to fear sleep in the meantime.

17. C: All of the statements listed in the question are true except for C. The chin EMG is actually often lower than it was seen in stage N2 when N3 sets in. The reason for this is stage N3 is a deeper stage of sleep, and the muscles relax even more than they had in stage N2 or N1 that preceded it.

18. D: Although most of the paste used in sleep labs is nontoxic, every single "Safety Data Sheet" for conductive pastes clearly states that the paste should be removed from the patient following use. Even if a patient is going to take a shower immediately, the paste should be wiped clean before the conclusion of the equipment-removal process in the morning.

19. A: An increase in chin EMG amplitude is only required in stage REM sleep. While most arousals will have an increase in muscle tone, the scoring guidelines of the American Academy of Sleep Medicine do not require it for NREM sleep stages. In REM, all of the same requirements apply in addition to the associated increase in the chin EMG.

20. C: All sensors that touch the patient's skin anywhere on the body are to be cleaned and disinfected. Sensors used in the nose and mouth require a higher level of disinfection than other sensors, which may only come into coincidental contact with the skin. The technician should always follow lab protocol for specific disinfection requirements on a case-by-case basis.

21. D: A minimum duration of 0.5 seconds and a maximum duration of 10 seconds are in line with scoring guidelines of the American Academy of Sleep Medicine (AASM), as are the criteria for the ending of a leg movement event. However the opposite is true for leg movements associated with respiratory events. According to the scoring guidelines of the AASM, leg movements associated with respiratory events are not scored because their causality is uncertain.

22. B: Since a hypopnea is a partial airway obstruction and not just the cessation of airflow like an obstructive apnea, it must be measured with volume or pressure. Thermal sensors measure the temperature and use the warmth of breath to measure the wax and waning of breaths. Pressure transducers measure the volume of the air being moved, so that when the airway is partially cut off, the technician can see that full breaths are not being taken. Scoring guidelines of the American Academy of Sleep Medicine require a specific reduction in the pressure transducer channel; the thermal sensor lacks the technology and sensitivity to detect those reductions.

23. B: According to the Clinical Guidelines for the Manual Titration of Positive Airway Pressure in Patients with Obstructive Sleep Apnea, pediatric patients under the age of 12 years should not have their PAP pressures raised above 15 cm. This consensus is based on physical tolerance and patient compliance studies. As far as compliance goes, if a patient will not use the CPAP at uncomfortable pressures, then it will not help them.

24. C: During REM, the body paralyzes the control of muscles to protect people from hurting themselves during active dreams. The chemical that is released during REM can usually be attributed to sleep paralysis when sleep is suddenly disrupted. Patients who are capable of moving and who have muscle tone during REM suffer from REM behavior disorder.

25. C: The recommendation of the American Academy of Sleep Medicine applies to patients in the sleep lab for a PAP study and those in the lab for a split-night study. Any time the technician suspects a patient might qualify for a split night, these processes should be resolved before beginning the study.

26. A: There is no maximum time limit for how long an obstructive apneic event can be. There are guidelines for resuming normal breath or resaturations of 2% or more defining the end of an event, but there is no hard cap on how long those events can be to qualify for scoring criteria.

27. A: The tape measure is placed with zero at FPz and lined up with all 10% up markings, including the 10% up from nasion and inion, until it wraps back around to FPz. Any other placement of the tape measure during circumference markings will yield incorrect results.

28. C: Patients who are left on suboptimal pressures will continue to under breathe and fail to get sufficient oxygen exchange to the heart. Even if a patient is not having specific or frequent events, CPAP should be used to increase the fullness of the flow wave and proper oxygenation of the blood.

29. D: Different machines and masks have charts for what is considered an acceptable clinical leak, when a therapeutic amount of pressure is still being delivered to the patient. For patients who are oral venting or are unable to keep the mask in place, a therapeutic leak range is acceptable only as long as it is not causing the patient to wake frequently.

30. C: Due to the pressure delivered through the nasal passages, nasal congestion can become a large problem with ongoing CPAP use. Water chambers and heated humidity exist to help lessen the impact PAP pressures may have on the nasal passages during use. Eye dryness and pain should only occur if the mask is not fitting properly. Dizziness and tinnitus are not side effects that patients could suffer from CPAP use, proper or otherwise.

31. D: Damaged equipment is one of the most common reasons patients begin suffering from sleep apnea during CPAP therapy use. Patients may not take care of their equipment, or it may be faulty. Usually this is the first thing that should be checked before moving forward with other possible issues. Excessive alcohol use has a negative effect on the patency of the upper airway. A pressure that was found to be optimal while a patient was sober in the sleep lab may not be sufficient to eliminate events for a patient who is drinking before bedtime at home.

32. B: The HFF, or high frequency filter, is used to adjust the rise time of a signal. The higher this filter is set the faster the signal wave will rise. The LFF is used to adjust the time constant, or fall time. Gain and sensitivity mean the same thing and will not affect the shape of the wave, only the size of the signal display.

33. C: The O1 lead is on the left side of the head, 20% of the total circumference of the head behind the T3 lead. The O2 lead is on the right side of the head, 20% of the total circumference of the head behind the T4 lead. An easy way to remember which side of the head a lead is on is to remember that odd numbered leads are on the left (e.g., O1, C3, T3) and even numbered leads are on the right (e.g., O2, C4, T4).

34. D: Frequency, or the number of times a wave occurs, is measured in Hertz, or cycles per second. This is the number of times a wave will repeat itself in one second. Voltage is measured in volts, and in polysomnography, in microvolts (uV). Amplitude is a measure of the height of a wave; therefore the more microvolts, the bigger the wave.

35. A: Sensitivity is measured in microvolts per millimeter, or uV/mm. What this means is that for each microvolt of a wave, the display will measure it in one mm. This also means that the larger the number of microvolts per millimeter, the smaller the wave will be displayed, because it will take more voltage to change the signal.

36. C: Generally the sensitivity is set between 5 uV/mm and 9 uV/mm. Of those choices 7 uV/mm would be the best answer. Normally, 1 uV/mm or 3 uV/mm would be far too high of a sensitivity setting (the lower the number of microvolts the less it will take to increase the wave size) and 15 uV/mm would be too low of a sensitivity setting (the higher the number of microvolts the more it will take to increase the wave size).

37. C: PLMS (periodic limb movements in sleep) is defined as at least 4 individual movements, 5 to 90 seconds apart, and each movement must last between 0.5 and 10 seconds. Remember that the patient must be asleep for PLMS. If there are leg movements when the patient is awake then it could be restless legs syndrome.

38. B: Sleep spindles are generally associated with stage 2 sleep. They are 12–14 Hz bursts of activity that have no amplitude requirement. Sleep spindles are also sometimes seen in stage 3 sleep, but the presence of delta waves differentiates stage 3 from stage 2 sleep.

39. B: The total recording time is measured from "lights off" to "lights on." In this case, the TRT was 6 hours. To get that in minutes, you would multiply 6 by 60 and get 360 minutes. The total recording time is valuable for determining the sleep efficiency, or the percentage of time the patient was asleep during the recording period.

40. A: The total sleep time (TST) is determined by adding the NREM sleep time to the REM sleep time. In this case, it was 275 minutes, or a little over 4.5 hours. The total sleep time is valuable for determining the sleep efficiency, or the percentage of time the patient was asleep during a recording period, and also for determining the apnea-hypopnea index (AHI) or respiratory disturbance index (RDI) of the patient during the study.

41. D: The total wake time is gathered by subtracting the total sleep time from the total recording time (TRT– TST = TWT). In this case the answer is 85. The total wake time is valuable for determining the sleep efficiency, or the percentage of the total sleep time the patient was asleep during the study, and for helping to determine if the patient has insomnia or long awakenings during the night.

42. C: The sleep efficiency, or the percentage of the total recording time the patient was asleep, is gained by dividing the total sleep time by the total recording time (TST/TRT = SE). In this case it is roughly 76%. This is useful for comparison to the ideal sleep efficiency and can help determine if the patient's sleep architecture is fractured.

43. B: The percentage of REM sleep is found by dividing the amount of time of REM sleep by the total sleep time: 45/275 = ~16%. The percentage of REM sleep is useful in determining if a patient's sleep architecture is fractured and is also useful in calculating the patient's REM apnea-hypopnea index (AHI) or respiratory disturbance index (RDI).

44. D: The percentage of NREM (non-REM) sleep is found by dividing the amount of NREM sleep by the total sleep time: 230/275 = ~84%. The percentage of non-REM sleep is useful in determining if a patient's sleep architecture is fractured and is also useful in determining the patient's non-REM apnea-hypopnea index (AHI) or respiratory disturbance index (RDI).

45. A: The mean, or average, sleep latency is obtained by adding the sleep latency of all the naps and then dividing by the number of naps. In this case the sleep latency of all the naps adds up to 25 minutes and when divided by the number of naps, 5, the mean latency ends up being 5 minutes. A mean sleep latency below 5 minutes might indicate narcolepsy or hypersomnolence (excessive sleepiness).

46. B: The mode is the number that occurs the most times. The sleep latencies for these naps were 5 minutes, 4 minutes, 3 minutes, 4 minutes, and 9 minutes. The number 4 occurs the most times therefore that is the mode sleep latency. The mode sleep latency can help determine if a patient has excessive sleepiness (hypersomnolence) at certain times of the day.

47. B: The median sleep latency is found by putting the sleep latencies in numerical order and using the one that occurs in the middle. In this case, it is 4 minutes. The median sleep latency can help determine if a patient has narcolepsy or hypersomnolence.

48. B: The MWT, or maintenance of wakefulness test, is used to determine if a patient can stay awake in difficult circumstances. In a MSLT, or multiple sleep latency test, the patient tries to go to sleep. A NPSG, or nocturnal polysomnogram, is the standard overnight diagnostic test. A REM behavior disorder test is used to diagnose patients who might have a REM behavior disorder.

49. D: A hypnagogic jerk is a muscle spasm or sudden contraction that happens during the transition from wakefulness to sleep. It is also called a hypnic jerk, sleep start, or night start. People who experience hypnagogic jerks also sometimes report that they have a falling sensation before the jerk. People who have reported having hypnic jerks also alternately report having sleep paralysis at times as well.

50. C: Raising the CPAP pressure is normally the best way to treat primary snoring if there are no mask leaks and no central apneas. Switching to BiPAP is done if the patient starts to develop central apneas. A mask leak might be causing problems with the treatment and preventing the tech from determining if a pressure is at a good therapeutic level.

51. B: At higher pressures CPAP can begin causing central apneas. The brain is responding to the excess air pressure by stopping respiration in order to keep rhythm with the normal gas exchange. If the apneas were obstructive in nature or if there are hypopneas or snoring, then the CPAP pressure is too low.

52. A: BiPAP S/T stands for bilevel positive airway pressure spontaneous/timed. It is used to treat central sleep apnea by providing two pressures, an IPAP (inspiratory positive airway pressure) and an EPAP (expiratory positive airway pressure), as well as a backup rate that will deliver a spontaneous, timed breath to the patient. The IPAP is normally 4–8 cwp higher than the EPAP and the backup rate is normally set at 8–12 breaths per minute (BPM).

53. D: Either decreasing the HFF (high frequency filter) or moving the affected electrode and repositioning it can eliminate muscle artifact. The LFF (low frequency filter) is used to filter out slower waves and would not have that much of an effect on muscle artifact. In general repositioning or re-applying leads is the best solution for dealing with artifacts, as changing the settings runs the risk of filtering out signals the technician may need.

54. A: Sweat artifact will look like slow delta waves (it is sometimes called "slow-wave artifact") and is caused by excessive sweat from a patient. The salt in the patient's sweat creates a chemical reaction in the electrodes that produce these slow waves. Sweat artifact normally affects the EEG and EOG channels. Even though these waves can be mistaken for delta waves, they are slower and will all move together. It is best corrected by drying the patient and adding a fan in the room, though adjusting the LFF may also eliminate this artifact.

55. B: Adjusting the filters is often the easiest way to eliminate artifact, but it can sometimes obscure signals that the technician may need to see. The best solution for eliminating artifact is to go to the source and reapply and replace the electrodes. Adjusting the filters should be used only if the patient is asleep and you do not wish to disturb her.

56. B: K-complexes, along with sleep spindles, are associated with stage 2 sleep. K-complexes are a sharp upward deflection (negative wave) followed by a slow downward deflection (positive) that is at least 0.5 seconds long. There is no amplitude requirement for K-complexes so they can appear very short or very small on the screen.

57. C: Cataplexy is a loss of muscle tone that sometimes accompanies a strong emotion (laughter, anger, fear) and is a symptom of narcolepsy. Other symptoms of narcolepsy include sleep paralysis, early onset of REM sleep, and reduced sleep latency.

58. C: Central sleep apnea is caused by brain damage, congestive heart failure, stroke, or COPD. Obesity is generally a cause of obstructive sleep apnea. Other causes of obstructive sleep apnea can be obstructions in the throat and upper airways such as tonsils or adenoids or excess tissue in the soft palate, deviated septum, or an oversized jaw. Alcohol and smoking increase the severity of obstructive apnea as well.

59. A: People with obstructive sleep apnea have a higher incidence of heart attack, stroke, and hypertension. It is very important that people with sleep apnea seek out treatment, as it is not just their quality of life that is affected by this disease. Public awareness of this disease is growing and more people are seeking treatment due to the health risks of obstructive apnea.

60. A: Insomnia is the most common sleep disorder in the United States. Insomnia has many causes including sleep apnea, anxiety, poor sleep hygiene, and certain medications. Insomnia can be either transient (1 to several days), short term (several days to 3 weeks), or chronic (3 weeks or more). There are treatment options for insomnia depending on the cause.

61. A: Due to his weight, this patient most likely has obstructive sleep apnea. His headaches and daytime sleepiness are probably due to the oxygen deprivation during sleep. His insomnia may result from waking from stage 1 sleep early in the evening due to apnea events. The limb movements that his wife is reporting may be resulting from frequent arousals due to obstructive apnea. A polysomnogram should be scheduled to confirm this diagnosis.

62. D: Switching to BiPAP will sometimes help the patient deal with higher pressures. The EPAP should be 4–8 cm lower than the IPAP pressure and should be set at a pressure where the apneas are cleared. The higher IPAP pressure should be set where the snoring and hypopneas have been cleared. The two different pressures will help the patient relax and fall back to sleep but still provide a good point in which to continue the titration.

63. D: The key things to look for are increased chin EMG activity, muscle movements and obstructive apneas in REM. This is abnormal and potentially dangerous to the patient or his bed partner. REM behavior disorder montages normally have a full EEG hookup, the standard baseline montage, and extra EMG leads on the arms to look for this activity. There should also be audio and video monitoring to look for any excess movements or activity in REM.

64. B: REM behavior disorder is often treated with benzodiazepines, clonidine, or Sinemet to prevent muscle activity during REM. Sleeping aids such as Ambien, Sonata, or Lunesta could potentially make the disorder worse as they are powerful narcoleptics. Medications such as Provigil, Ritalin, or Dexedrine are stimulants that are often used to treat narcolepsy.

65. C: Modafinil (Provigil), methylphenidate (Ritalin), dextroamphetamine (Dexedrine), pemoline (Cylert), and methamphetamines are powerful stimulants used to treat narcolepsy. Ambien is used to treat insomnia and Mirapex is used to treat PLMS. These drugs prevent the sleepiness associated with narcolepsy and are used in conjunction with REM-suppressing drugs to prevent cataplexy, hypnagogic hallucinations, and sleep. In the past certain antidepressants were used to treat narcolepsy as well. These drugs can be very dangerous and the patient should be followed closely by the prescribing physician.

66. B: The technician should not give information on the results of the study to the patient. This is the duty of the doctor, and the technician is not qualified to make an interpretation on her own. The technician is responsible for making sure the patient is safe and as comfortable as possible, conducting the study accurately, maintaining the equipment, and making notes for the doctor and scoring technician.

67. C: Different labs have different policies and systems for patient acquisition, but in general the patient's name, date of birth, gender, referring doctor, and the study identification number are all logged in before the beginning of the study. Other things that may also be included are the patient's height and weight, his insurance, his social security number, his medication, and the study type.

68. D: Most major antidepressant medications such as SSRIs (selective serotonin reuptake inhibitors), TCAs (tricyclic antidepressants) and MAOIs (monoamine oxidase inhibitors) have been proven to suppress REM sleep and delay REM onset. Also, antidepressants can cause daytime sleepiness and conversely insomnia in some patients. Trimipramine, mirtazapine and nefazodone are the only antidepressant medications that do not suppress REM sleep and in some cases may actually increase REM activity.

69. B: Alcohol can suppress slow-wave stage 3 sleep and REM sleep. Moderate levels of alcohol can cause sleepiness and may extend sleep for a longer time, but high levels of blood alcohol can cause insomnia and sleep fragmentation. Chronic alcoholism can completely suppress both delta-wave stage 3 sleep and REM sleep and cause chronic insomnia.

70. A: Nicotine, not necessarily just from smoking but also from the nicotine patch and nicotine gum, is a stimulant that may cause insomnia. Smoking may result in a worsening of apnea as the damage done to the lungs and airways may result in upper airway resistance and low blood oxygen saturation.

71. B: In the EKG the first wave in a heartbeat is the P wave. The P wave represents the atrial contraction. The period after the last heartbeat and the P wave is the sinus node impulse; during this period the atrium of the heart is filling with blood. After the atrial contraction the blood fills the ventricles to be pumped out of the heart.

72. C: In an electrocardiogram (ECG or EKG) the QRS complex represents ventricular contraction, which is when the ventricles pump blood out of the heart. Each QRS complex lasts from 0.04 to 0.10 seconds. The period after a QRS complex (the ST segment) is when the ventricles begin to repolarize.

73. B: The T wave represents ventricular repolarization in an EKG. When the ventricles repolarize it concludes the heartbeat and sets the stage for the next heartbeat. In all, it takes less than a second for the heart to go through the contraction-relaxation cycle and produce a heartbeat. A normal adult's heart beats at 60–100 beats per minute. A slower heart rate is referred to as bradycardia and a faster heart rate is tachycardia.

74. C: In a differential amplifier, the type of amplifier used in polysomnography, G1 represents the first signal input, or exploring electrode, while G2 represents the second signal input, or the reference electrode. The difference in the voltage that these two electrodes are picking up produces the signal seen on the screen. For example, in the EEG the C3 lead is the G1, exploring electrode, while the A2 lead is the G2, reference electrode; this is why that channel is labeled C3/A2.

75. A: The minimum AHI (apnea-hypopnea index) to be diagnosed with OSA (obstructive sleep apnea) and qualify for CPAP is 5/hr. An AHI below 5/hr may lead to a diagnosis of upper airway

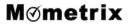

resistance syndrome or no diagnosis at all, but most insurance companies will not authorize an overnight CPAP study, much less a CPAP machine, with an AHI of less than 5/hr.

How to Overcome Test Anxiety

Just the thought of taking a test is enough to make most people a little nervous. A test is an important event that can have a long-term impact on your future, so it's important to take it seriously and it's natural to feel anxious about performing well. But just because anxiety is normal, that doesn't mean that it's helpful in test taking, or that you should simply accept it as part of your life. Anxiety can have a variety of effects. These effects can be mild, like making you feel slightly nervous, or severe, like blocking your ability to focus or remember even a simple detail.

If you experience test anxiety—whether severe or mild—it's important to know how to beat it. To discover this, first you need to understand what causes test anxiety.

Causes of Test Anxiety

While we often think of anxiety as an uncontrollable emotional state, it can actually be caused by simple, practical things. One of the most common causes of test anxiety is that a person does not feel adequately prepared for their test. This feeling can be the result of many different issues such as poor study habits or lack of organization, but the most common culprit is time management. Starting to study too late, failing to organize your study time to cover all of the material, or being distracted while you study will mean that you're not well prepared for the test. This may lead to cramming the night before, which will cause you to be physically and mentally exhausted for the test. Poor time management also contributes to feelings of stress, fear, and hopelessness as you realize you are not well prepared but don't know what to do about it.

Other times, test anxiety is not related to your preparation for the test but comes from unresolved fear. This may be a past failure on a test, or poor performance on tests in general. It may come from comparing yourself to others who seem to be performing better or from the stress of living up to expectations. Anxiety may be driven by fears of the future—how failure on this test would affect your educational and career goals. These fears are often completely irrational, but they can still negatively impact your test performance.

> **Review Video: 3 Reasons You Have Test Anxiety**
> Visit mometrix.com/academy and enter code: 428468

Elements of Test Anxiety

As mentioned earlier, test anxiety is considered to be an emotional state, but it has physical and mental components as well. Sometimes you may not even realize that you are suffering from test anxiety until you notice the physical symptoms. These can include trembling hands, rapid heartbeat, sweating, nausea, and tense muscles. Extreme anxiety may lead to fainting or vomiting. Obviously, any of these symptoms can have a negative impact on testing. It is important to recognize them as soon as they begin to occur so that you can address the problem before it damages your performance.

> **Review Video: 3 Ways to Tell You Have Test Anxiety**
> Visit mometrix.com/academy and enter code: 927847

The mental components of test anxiety include trouble focusing and inability to remember learned information. During a test, your mind is on high alert, which can help you recall information and stay focused for an extended period of time. However, anxiety interferes with your mind's natural processes, causing you to blank out, even on the questions you know well. The strain of testing during anxiety makes it difficult to stay focused, especially on a test that may take several hours. Extreme anxiety can take a huge mental toll, making it difficult not only to recall test information but even to understand the test questions or pull your thoughts together.

> **Review Video: How Test Anxiety Affects Memory**
> Visit mometrix.com/academy and enter code: 609003

Effects of Test Anxiety

Test anxiety is like a disease—if left untreated, it will get progressively worse. Anxiety leads to poor performance, and this reinforces the feelings of fear and failure, which in turn lead to poor performances on subsequent tests. It can grow from a mild nervousness to a crippling condition. If allowed to progress, test anxiety can have a big impact on your schooling, and consequently on your future.

Test anxiety can spread to other parts of your life. Anxiety on tests can become anxiety in any stressful situation, and blanking on a test can turn into panicking in a job situation. But fortunately, you don't have to let anxiety rule your testing and determine your grades. There are a number of relatively simple steps you can take to move past anxiety and function normally on a test and in the rest of life.

> **Review Video: How Test Anxiety Impacts Your Grades**
> Visit mometrix.com/academy and enter code: 939819

Physical Steps for Beating Test Anxiety

While test anxiety is a serious problem, the good news is that it can be overcome. It doesn't have to control your ability to think and remember information. While it may take time, you can begin taking steps today to beat anxiety.

Just as your first hint that you may be struggling with anxiety comes from the physical symptoms, the first step to treating it is also physical. Rest is crucial for having a clear, strong mind. If you are tired, it is much easier to give in to anxiety. But if you establish good sleep habits, your body and mind will be ready to perform optimally, without the strain of exhaustion. Additionally, sleeping well helps you to retain information better, so you're more likely to recall the answers when you see the test questions.

Getting good sleep means more than going to bed on time. It's important to allow your brain time to relax. Take study breaks from time to time so it doesn't get overworked, and don't study right before bed. Take time to rest your mind before trying to rest your body, or you may find it difficult to fall asleep.

> **Review Video: The Importance of Sleep for Your Brain**
> Visit mometrix.com/academy and enter code: 319338

Along with sleep, other aspects of physical health are important in preparing for a test. Good nutrition is vital for good brain function. Sugary foods and drinks may give a burst of energy but this burst is followed by a crash, both physically and emotionally. Instead, fuel your body with protein and vitamin-rich foods.

Also, drink plenty of water. Dehydration can lead to headaches and exhaustion, especially if your brain is already under stress from the rigors of the test. Particularly if your test is a long one, drink water during the breaks. And if possible, take an energy-boosting snack to eat between sections.

> **Review Video: How Diet Can Affect your Mood**
> Visit mometrix.com/academy and enter code: 624317

Along with sleep and diet, a third important part of physical health is exercise. Maintaining a steady workout schedule is helpful, but even taking 5-minute study breaks to walk can help get your blood pumping faster and clear your head. Exercise also releases endorphins, which contribute to a positive feeling and can help combat test anxiety.

When you nurture your physical health, you are also contributing to your mental health. If your body is healthy, your mind is much more likely to be healthy as well. So take time to rest, nourish your body with healthy food and water, and get moving as much as possible. Taking these physical steps will make you stronger and more able to take the mental steps necessary to overcome test anxiety.

Mental Steps for Beating Test Anxiety

Working on the mental side of test anxiety can be more challenging, but as with the physical side, there are clear steps you can take to overcome it. As mentioned earlier, test anxiety often stems from lack of preparation, so the obvious solution is to prepare for the test. Effective studying may be the most important weapon you have for beating test anxiety, but you can and should employ several other mental tools to combat fear.

First, boost your confidence by reminding yourself of past success—tests or projects that you aced. If you're putting as much effort into preparing for this test as you did for those, there's no reason you should expect to fail here. Work hard to prepare; then trust your preparation.

Second, surround yourself with encouraging people. It can be helpful to find a study group, but be sure that the people you're around will encourage a positive attitude. If you spend time with others who are anxious or cynical, this will only contribute to your own anxiety. Look for others who are motivated to study hard from a desire to succeed, not from a fear of failure.

Third, reward yourself. A test is physically and mentally tiring, even without anxiety, and it can be helpful to have something to look forward to. Plan an activity following the test, regardless of the outcome, such as going to a movie or getting ice cream.

When you are taking the test, if you find yourself beginning to feel anxious, remind yourself that you know the material. Visualize successfully completing the test. Then take a few deep, relaxing breaths and return to it. Work through the questions carefully but with confidence, knowing that you are capable of succeeding.

Developing a healthy mental approach to test taking will also aid in other areas of life. Test anxiety affects more than just the actual test—it can be damaging to your mental health and even contribute to depression. It's important to beat test anxiety before it becomes a problem for more than testing.

> **Review Video: Test Anxiety and Depression**
> Visit mometrix.com/academy and enter code: 904704

Study Strategy

Being prepared for the test is necessary to combat anxiety, but what does being prepared look like? You may study for hours on end and still not feel prepared. What you need is a strategy for test prep. The next few pages outline our recommended steps to help you plan out and conquer the challenge of preparation.

STEP 1: SCOPE OUT THE TEST

Learn everything you can about the format (multiple choice, essay, etc.) and what will be on the test. Gather any study materials, course outlines, or sample exams that may be available. Not only will this help you to prepare, but knowing what to expect can help to alleviate test anxiety.

STEP 2: MAP OUT THE MATERIAL

Look through the textbook or study guide and make note of how many chapters or sections it has. Then divide these over the time you have. For example, if a book has 15 chapters and you have five days to study, you need to cover three chapters each day. Even better, if you have the time, leave an extra day at the end for overall review after you have gone through the material in depth.

If time is limited, you may need to prioritize the material. Look through it and make note of which sections you think you already have a good grasp on, and which need review. While you are studying, skim quickly through the familiar sections and take more time on the challenging parts. Write out your plan so you don't get lost as you go. Having a written plan also helps you feel more in control of the study, so anxiety is less likely to arise from feeling overwhelmed at the amount to cover.

STEP 3: GATHER YOUR TOOLS

Decide what study method works best for you. Do you prefer to highlight in the book as you study and then go back over the highlighted portions? Or do you type out notes of the important information? Or is it helpful to make flashcards that you can carry with you? Assemble the pens, index cards, highlighters, post-it notes, and any other materials you may need so you won't be distracted by getting up to find things while you study.

If you're having a hard time retaining the information or organizing your notes, experiment with different methods. For example, try color-coding by subject with colored pens, highlighters, or post-it notes. If you learn better by hearing, try recording yourself reading your notes so you can listen while in the car, working out, or simply sitting at your desk. Ask a friend to quiz you from your flashcards, or try teaching someone the material to solidify it in your mind.

STEP 4: CREATE YOUR ENVIRONMENT

It's important to avoid distractions while you study. This includes both the obvious distractions like visitors and the subtle distractions like an uncomfortable chair (or a too-comfortable couch that makes you want to fall asleep). Set up the best study environment possible: good lighting and a comfortable work area. If background music helps you focus, you may want to turn it on, but otherwise keep the room quiet. If you are using a computer to take notes, be sure you don't have any other windows open, especially applications like social media, games, or anything else that could distract you. Silence your phone and turn off notifications. Be sure to keep water close by so you stay hydrated while you study (but avoid unhealthy drinks and snacks).

Also, take into account the best time of day to study. Are you freshest first thing in the morning? Try to set aside some time then to work through the material. Is your mind clearer in the afternoon or evening? Schedule your study session then. Another method is to study at the same time of day that you will take the test, so that your brain gets used to working on the material at that time and will be ready to focus at test time.

STEP 5: STUDY!

Once you have done all the study preparation, it's time to settle into the actual studying. Sit down, take a few moments to settle your mind so you can focus, and begin to follow your study plan. Don't give in to distractions or let yourself procrastinate. This is your time to prepare so you'll be ready to fearlessly approach the test. Make the most of the time and stay focused.

Of course, you don't want to burn out. If you study too long you may find that you're not retaining the information very well. Take regular study breaks. For example, taking five minutes out of every hour to walk briskly, breathing deeply and swinging your arms, can help your mind stay fresh.

As you get to the end of each chapter or section, it's a good idea to do a quick review. Remind yourself of what you learned and work on any difficult parts. When you feel that you've mastered the material, move on to the next part. At the end of your study session, briefly skim through your notes again.

But while review is helpful, cramming last minute is NOT. If at all possible, work ahead so that you won't need to fit all your study into the last day. Cramming overloads your brain with more information than it can process and retain, and your tired mind may struggle to recall even previously learned information when it is overwhelmed with last-minute study. Also, the urgent nature of cramming and the stress placed on your brain contribute to anxiety. You'll be more likely to go to the test feeling unprepared and having trouble thinking clearly.

So don't cram, and don't stay up late before the test, even just to review your notes at a leisurely pace. Your brain needs rest more than it needs to go over the information again. In fact, plan to finish your studies by noon or early afternoon the day before the test. Give your brain the rest of the day to relax or focus on other things, and get a good night's sleep. Then you will be fresh for the test and better able to recall what you've studied.

STEP 6: TAKE A PRACTICE TEST

Many courses offer sample tests, either online or in the study materials. This is an excellent resource to check whether you have mastered the material, as well as to prepare for the test format and environment.

Check the test format ahead of time: the number of questions, the type (multiple choice, free response, etc.), and the time limit. Then create a plan for working through them. For example, if you have 30 minutes to take a 60-question test, your limit is 30 seconds per question. Spend less time on the questions you know well so that you can take more time on the difficult ones.

If you have time to take several practice tests, take the first one open book, with no time limit. Work through the questions at your own pace and make sure you fully understand them. Gradually work up to taking a test under test conditions: sit at a desk with all study materials put away and set a timer. Pace yourself to make sure you finish the test with time to spare and go back to check your answers if you have time.

After each test, check your answers. On the questions you missed, be sure you understand why you missed them. Did you misread the question (tests can use tricky wording)? Did you forget the information? Or was it something you hadn't learned? Go back and study any shaky areas that the practice tests reveal.

Taking these tests not only helps with your grade, but also aids in combating test anxiety. If you're already used to the test conditions, you're less likely to worry about it, and working through tests until you're scoring well gives you a confidence boost. Go through the practice tests until you feel comfortable, and then you can go into the test knowing that you're ready for it.

Test Tips

On test day, you should be confident, knowing that you've prepared well and are ready to answer the questions. But aside from preparation, there are several test day strategies you can employ to maximize your performance.

First, as stated before, get a good night's sleep the night before the test (and for several nights before that, if possible). Go into the test with a fresh, alert mind rather than staying up late to study.

Try not to change too much about your normal routine on the day of the test. It's important to eat a nutritious breakfast, but if you normally don't eat breakfast at all, consider eating just a protein bar. If you're a coffee drinker, go ahead and have your normal coffee. Just make sure you time it so that the caffeine doesn't wear off right in the middle of your test. Avoid sugary beverages, and drink enough water to stay hydrated but not so much that you need a restroom break 10 minutes into the test. If your test isn't first thing in the morning, consider going for a walk or doing a light workout before the test to get your blood flowing.

Allow yourself enough time to get ready, and leave for the test with plenty of time to spare so you won't have the anxiety of scrambling to arrive in time. Another reason to be early is to select a good seat. It's helpful to sit away from doors and windows, which can be distracting. Find a good seat, get out your supplies, and settle your mind before the test begins.

When the test begins, start by going over the instructions carefully, even if you already know what to expect. Make sure you avoid any careless mistakes by following the directions.

Then begin working through the questions, pacing yourself as you've practiced. If you're not sure on an answer, don't spend too much time on it, and don't let it shake your confidence. Either skip it and come back later, or eliminate as many wrong answers as possible and guess among the remaining ones. Don't dwell on these questions as you continue—put them out of your mind and focus on what lies ahead.

Be sure to read all of the answer choices, even if you're sure the first one is the right answer. Sometimes you'll find a better one if you keep reading. But don't second-guess yourself if you do immediately know the answer. Your gut instinct is usually right. Don't let test anxiety rob you of the information you know.

If you have time at the end of the test (and if the test format allows), go back and review your answers. Be cautious about changing any, since your first instinct tends to be correct, but make sure you didn't misread any of the questions or accidentally mark the wrong answer choice. Look over any you skipped and make an educated guess.

At the end, leave the test feeling confident. You've done your best, so don't waste time worrying about your performance or wishing you could change anything. Instead, celebrate the successful

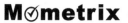

completion of this test. And finally, use this test to learn how to deal with anxiety even better next time.

> **Review Video: 5 Tips to Beat Test Anxiety**
> Visit mometrix.com/academy and enter code: 570656

Important Qualification

Not all anxiety is created equal. If your test anxiety is causing major issues in your life beyond the classroom or testing center, or if you are experiencing troubling physical symptoms related to your anxiety, it may be a sign of a serious physiological or psychological condition. If this sounds like your situation, we strongly encourage you to seek professional help.

Thank You

We at Mometrix would like to extend our heartfelt thanks to you, our friend and patron, for allowing us to play a part in your journey. It is a privilege to serve people from all walks of life who are unified in their commitment to building the best future they can for themselves.

The preparation you devote to these important testing milestones may be the most valuable educational opportunity you have for making a real difference in your life. We encourage you to put your heart into it—that feeling of succeeding, overcoming, and yes, conquering will be well worth the hours you've invested.

We want to hear your story, your struggles and your successes, and if you see any opportunities for us to improve our materials so we can help others even more effectively in the future, please share that with us as well. **The team at Mometrix would be absolutely thrilled to hear from you!** So please, send us an email (support@mometrix.com) and let's stay in touch.

> **If you'd like some additional help, check out these other resources we offer for your exam:**
> **http://mometrixflashcards.com/RPSGT**

Additional Bonus Material

Due to our efforts to try to keep this book to a manageable length, we've created a link that will give you access to all of your additional bonus material:

mometrix.com/bonus948/cpsgt